"I have worked with Laura Keegan for nearly 20 years. Since her consultations with breastfeeding families are necessarily private, I never knew the secret(s) that made her patients so fiercely loyal and grateful. Well, here they are. Using beautiful images and clear, simple, accurate descriptions, Laura has created a manual of wisdom and celebration that should be read by anyone who is, has, or is going to breastfeed an infant."

—Larry Baskind, MD, FAAP

"Working with Laura Keegan in my busy pediatric practice for the past 15 years, I have had the opportunity to witness firsthand her excellence as a clinician and her caring compassionate heart. I have been referring mothers to her for breastfeeding consultation and have witnessed literally hundreds of children benefiting from her wisdom. Her ability to simplify and communicate what is all too often over-complicated in our culture is reflected in the long-lasting relationships she develops with her patients. I am so pleased that this is reflected in the pages of this book and look forward to recommending it to new mothers."

—Stephen Cowan, MD, FAAP

I received Laura Keegan's book shortly before the birth of my twin girls. I had so much trouble beginning breastfeeding with my firstborn. I had a lot of pain and frequent nursing despite the help of specialists. I was hoping things would be different with my twins. However, there were new challenges: both babies were placed in the NICU after an unexpected Cesarean birth, and one of the babies was bottle-fed for 3 days while we were separated. Soon after the births, I opened the book on my hospital bed and read it over and over between feeds with the daughter who was with me and referred to it while I was trying to latch her on. I absorbed all the steps and tried until I knew we got it right. When my other daughter returned, I successfully latched on both babies using what I'd learned and practiced from the book. Before this experience, I never would have believed that learning the correct latch in this book meant that I would spend less time nursing my twins than I did nursing my firstborn and without the pain of sore nipples. After the birth of my fourth child, I needed to refer to the book to achieve the correct latch again. Take the time to study this book. Read and reread it carefully; look at the photographs and keep the book accessible. It is worth the time and effort."

—Mary P. Anderson, mother of four

"I am a breastfeeding mother of twins. During the first two months of my son's life, he was a slow weight gainer. I tried several different techniques that I had read about in other books, but none of them seemed to be working. After only one session with Laura Keegan in which she helped me make the slightest adjustment in how my son was latching on, Omar-Sol started gaining weight by leaps and bounds!!! I am happy to report that one year later, my children are happily breastfeeding and growing wonderfully. All that Laura taught me and more is beautifully photographed and clearly described in these pages. This book is a must read!!"

—Marla Teyolia, MSW and Author *Empowered Mama: a Modern Stay at Home Mom's Guide to Activism, Leadership, and Living a Passion-filled Life*

"I am thrilled that there finally is a book that will simplify breastfeeding and show us the way mother nature intended it to be. As a mother of two, my experiences differ vastly. The first was filled with anxiety, engorgement, mastitis and cracked nipples. The thought of formula feeding even entered my mind. Second time around Laura Keegan showed me how to latch my baby on properly. It amazed me how right it felt and, as a result, I didn't have any of the problems I had with my first. Working as a doula, I am excited to share this book with my clients. I have referred many women to Laura and they all share my enthusiasm and gratitude for her deep understanding of the subject. This book is for women who want to discover the JOY of breastfeeding."

—Rebecka Danielsson DeRoche, Doula

"I was unable to breastfeed my son for 6 weeks, despite having no problems with my firstborn. I was told by specialists that my baby had an abnormal suck and that I had an inverted nipple on one side. I fed him my pumped breastmilk with a bottle after first attempting to nurse him at the breast at every feed. When my son was 6 weeks old, my aunt, Jane Nienstadt, showed me a technique that she had learned from Laura Keegan. I was finally able to get my son to latch on and nurse. I was so excited! I was relieved that my son could feed at the breast and did not have an abnormal suck. He continued to nurse for 17 months without any difficulty."

—Nancy Vilander

"Laura Keegan's soft spoken assurance that mothers can breastfeed their babies successfully and comfortably is the gift she's given to countless families. That message is clear in this lovely book, but it's most useful element is the practical information which cuts through much of the rhetoric in the lactation press. Mothers will be able to adjust positions, improve latches and solve other problems as they and their babies learn to feed."

—Mary Ellen Stavitz, MSN, CPNP

"Laura Keegan offers a nurturing self-help approach, which enables moms to embrace breast-feeding without fear. I have experienced the benefits from her work with my own newborn as well as my patients. As a pediatric cranial sacral therapist, I have witnessed how impacting it is for a newborn to latch and breastfeed successfully. When treating newborns with Laura, I see a far better scenario for these babies and their parents because of her self-healing approach and devotion to nature's intention. The beauty and simplicity of the natural techniques revealed in this book will facilitate your process. The education is a gift for our children and grandchildren."

—Anne Samojedny, PT, CST

"As a childbirth educator and postpartum doula I have seen women struggle with self doubt, fear and uncertainty. To a postpartum woman, the obstacles and challenges of breastfeeding can feel overwhelming and insurmountable, and can easily undermine confidence in all aspects of mother-hood. One of Laura Keegan's greatest gifts is in her ability to allow women to unveil for themselves the intuitive wisdom that lies buried beneath layers of self doubt. Her unique technique relies on paying close attention to the mother/baby dyad. It works… beautifully and simply. As a postpar-tum doula I have seen Laura's technique not only put an end to breastfeeding challenges, but also empower women to embrace their new role as a mother with confidence."

—Janet Donat, CCE, Doula

"This beautifully illustrated book will help the world see how breastfeeding should be seen... as love personified."

—Dr. Carol J Phillips author of *Hands of Love: Seven Steps to the Miracle of Birth*

"I can remember how excited I was to breastfeed my daughter Ella and yet how quickly my excitement turned into anxiety and stress. The nurses explained to me that they were uncertain how my body would respond (due to a past surgery). It was very unsettling and I kept losing my confidence. I was having trouble getting her on the breast and became very sore. Each time I tried, it became more uncomfortable. Then just as we were anticipating leaving and going home with our daughter, the doctor came in to tell us that she had some serious complications and she needed to be monitored. I was in shock. I couldn't believe it. Luckily she was able to stay at the hospital nursery and was placed on cardiac/respiratory monitoring. She was in an isolette and could not be with me. I walked into the nursery and there was my little girl hooked up to all these wires, machines and isolated all by herself. I was really scared and was ready to give up on breastfeeding from all the stress and feeling like I just wasn't getting it right. But I knew that it was what I wanted deep down, and how women have done this generation after generation. Why couldn't I get it? Every time I tried to feed her, it became worse and worse. My nipples were so sore and beginning to crack, and all this was compounded by the stress I felt because my daughter was not urinating enough. They began to cup feed her. I lost all hope and felt like a failure. I called my pediatrician who instantly said, 'You need Laura Keegan to come in and see you; she will help you get through this.' As soon as I spoke with Laura on the phone, she made me feel like I could do this. She came to the hospital and was my saving grace. Her patience, compassion and faith in me and my body gave me the confidence to stay with breastfeeding. She made me practice a few simple adjustments and there it was, I was breastfeeding without pain. It was the greatest gift I could give Ella while she was going through this. I was able to nurse her with all these tubes and wires and nurture my bond with her. I really feel that breastfeeding helped her move through her healing much easier. I had a lot of challenges and Laura's simple techniques helped me tremendously. Every fear and doubt dissolved and I knew if I kept with it, I could do this and I did. My daughter is now almost 15 months and I still nurse her and thanks to Laura she gave me the confidence I needed to breastfeed with ease and comfort."

—Anne E. West, RN, LAc (holistic nurse / acupuncturist)

Book orders and information:
www.lifeforcefamilyhealth.com
www.laurakeegan.com

Breastfeeding with Comfort and Joy

A Photographic Guide for Mom and Those Who Help Her

By Laura Keegan, R.N., F.N.P.

Text and photographs © 2008, Laura Keegan.

Foreword © 2008, Robert Schiller.

All rights reserved.

No part of this book may be reproduced in any manner without written permission from the copyright holder.

Design and layout: Jennifer Trail, Intrinsic Audio Visual / www.intrinsicaudiovisual.com

ISBN 978-0-615-19383-0

Published in the United States

Lifeforce Family Health Care

www.lifeforcefamilyhealth.com

www.laurakeegan.com

Printing: One World Press / www.oneworldpress.com

This book was printed in China on acid-free paper using soy ink.

This book is dedicated to parents and their babies.

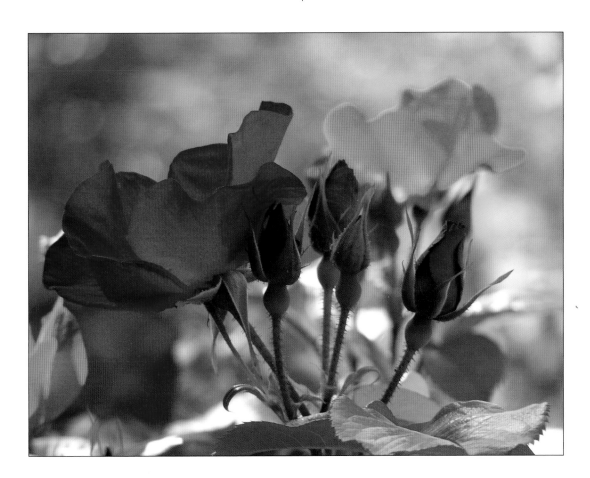

Contents

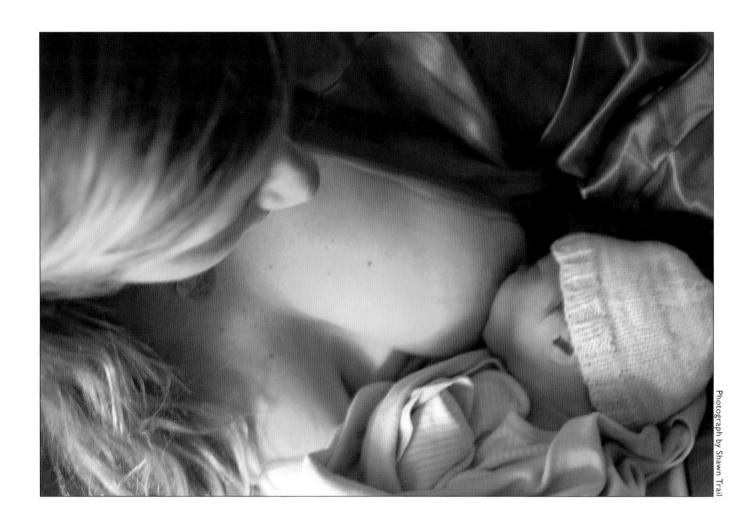

Foreword

Raising healthy children has become a daunting task for most parents. This process starts with their child's birth, with the mother providing the best nourishment for her baby. Our history and current research stress the obvious: healthier babies are breastfed babies. We don't need more studies to convince us of the merits of breastfeeding. We need help on how to promote successful breastfeeding, overcoming barriers, dispelling myths. We need intelligent, creative, supportive health educators, who understand the significant difficulties mothers face with breastfeeding their newborns, and offer simple, practical help.

Laura Keegan is the advocate and educator that we need, and her book is the guide. She has produced this extraordinary volume on the methods and attitudes to successful breastfeeding. She is committed to restoring breastfeeding to its proper place in raising a healthy child. Her extensive experience as a mother, nurse practitioner, health educator, and insightful motivator has provided her with a unique perspective on successful breastfeeding.

As a family physician practicing at a community health center in New York City for over 20 years, I have cared for numerous newborns and their parents, comprised from a diverse range of ethnic and social backgrounds. For parents in all families, establishing positive and constructive relationships with their children is crucial to raising a healthy child. For parents, the feeding of their newborn is a fundamental element of this evolving parent-child relationship. Successful breastfeeding can be an essential first step in promoting an optimal relationship. I see this book as an invaluable and essential resource for all breastfeeding mothers.

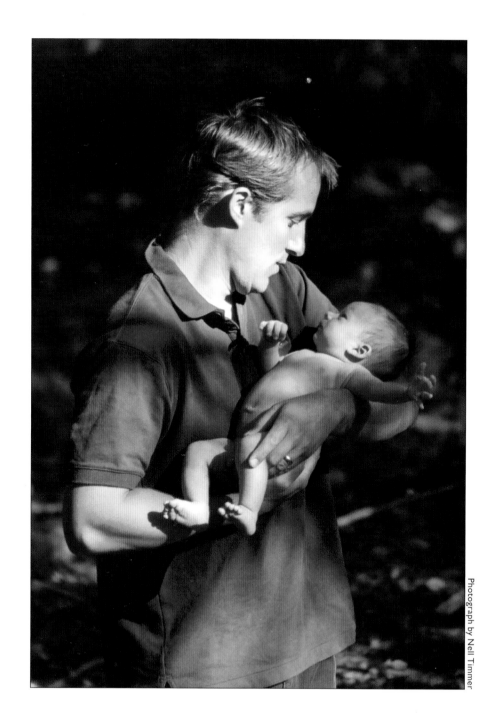

This book goes beyond the usual mechanics of breastfeeding. With clear and precise language, and stunning and instructive photographs, it conveys the ease, joy and pleasure of breastfeeding one's child. Laura describes in detail how to anticipate, prevent and overcome many of the common problems with breastfeeding. She has achieved a wonderful balance and openness, acknowledging the limitations of breastfeeding and the occasional need for bottle-feeding. As an advocate, Laura is encouraging all mothers to breastfeed, but more importantly she reminds us of the bigger picture. It is not how much mothers breastfeed, but how breastfeeding becomes part of their relationship with their child. The milk may flow easily or with difficulty; the child may be calm or fussy. Laura reassures us mothers and children will be fine.

Reading a book on breastfeeding may seem like reading a book on bike riding. There are so many things to master: pedaling, balance, steering, and speed. In fact, you really need a bike and have to get on it to learn. Breastfeeding is similar. You need your baby, but Laura's book brings you as close to the experience as a book can provide. Like a patient and supportive parent coaching a young rider, she is there with you, calming your fears, strengthening your confidence, and celebrating your joy.

I have had the pleasure of knowing Laura her entire career, including working together for a number of years in a group medical practice. She is an unusually gifted clinician and educator. She has produced a book as simple, beautiful, and nourishing as the act of breastfeeding itself.

Robert Schiller, MD

Chair, Alfred & Gail Englenberg Department of Family Medicine
  Beth Israel Medical Center, NY, NY
Senior VP of Clinical Affairs, Institute for Family Health, NY, NY
Assistant Professor Department of Family Medicine
  Albert Einstein College of Medicine, Bronx, NY

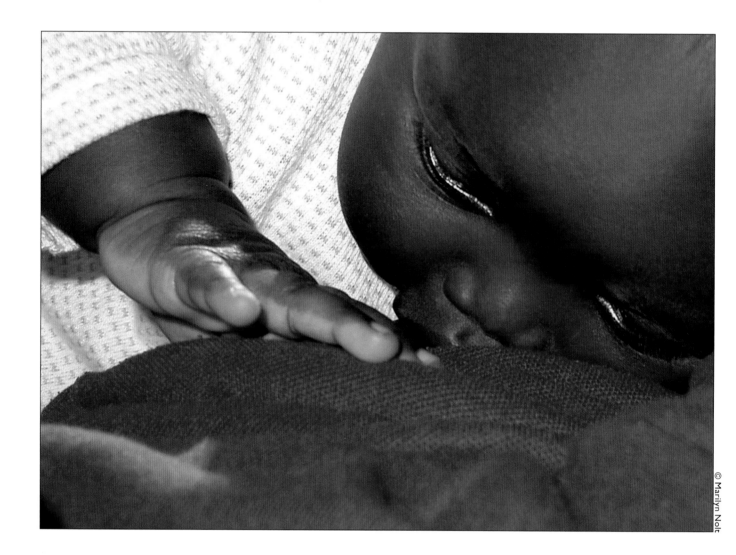

xx

Acknowledgments

I would like to acknowledge all the parents and babies I have worked with over the years. I have been honored to work with families during the most sacred of times as they bring new lives into the world and care for their infants. Most of what I know I have learned from these families. I am especially grateful to the families who allowed me to photograph them and allowed their images to grace the pages of this book: Erika Wood and Ronan Wood-Gallagher; Tanya Stepan and Robert, Isabel and Colin Murray; Mei-Sang Hsieh and Leon Brown; Rebecka Danielsson DeRoche and Allan and Lukas DeRoche; Debra Schaefer and Andrew and Michael Hoffart; Maria Stein Marrison and Anna Sofia Marrison; and Marla, Omar and Sophia Teyolia and William Teyolia Powers and Minerva Casillas.

The work of Mary Renfrew, Chloe Fisher and Suzanne Arms in their book *Bestfeeding: How to Breastfeed Your Baby* is used throughout this book to describe and illustrate proper position and latch. Chloe and Suzanne are two of my greatest teachers of breastfeeding. Chloe's conference presentations, videos, and communications with me over the years allowed me to incorporate her clinical knowledge and expertise successfully in my practice. Suzanne reviewed the first draft of this book and gave me the encouragement I needed to pursue the writing of a book.

Many people helped me to create a book from my writings and photographs. Erika Wood did the initial layout in 1999. Her work not only formed the foundation from which the book developed and grew but allowed me to distribute the book personally to help many women and their babies.

Jennifer Trail's work and eye for color and clarity allowed my photographs to be as true to life as possible. She has done the design and layout for this book and has followed me through many revisions.

Peggy Guyett has proofread many revisions of this book for me. I actually enjoyed this tedious process because she is a great teacher.

The first printing of this book was made possible, in part, by a grant awarded by The Eileen Fisher Foundation.

I am ever grateful to my husband, Kevin Keegan, who never wavered in his belief in my ability to grow, birth, and nourish all of my babies.

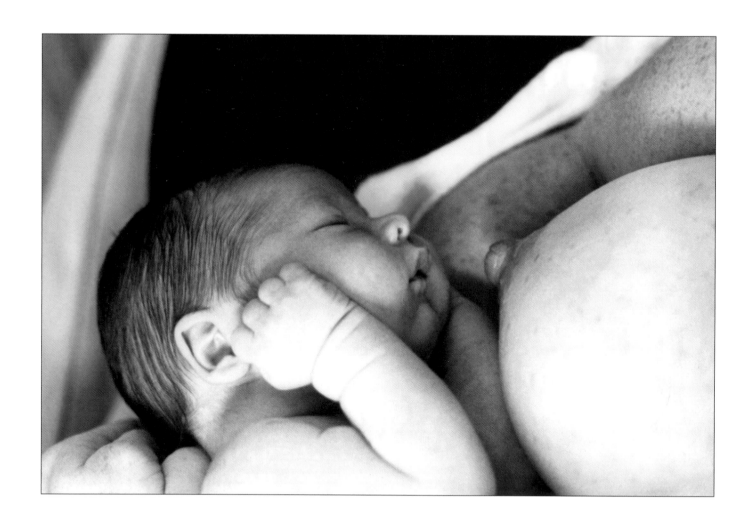

Preface : How to Use This Book

This book was meant to be read from cover to cover and then reread for details. Each section is important in terms of a description of what is helpful in the practicalities of feeding your baby. Just as important are explanations included to help you understand some of the subtle ways you and those around you can create the ideal environment for you and your baby to thrive together.

The book is full of pictures and meant to be read in its entirety in one sitting the first time you read it. If you have children or already have your baby, you may not be able to read the entire book without interruptions. It is still preferable to try to read through the book once at least from the introduction through the sections in the main body of the book, and to leave the appendices for when you have more time.

The sections entitled "Positioning," "Posture," "How You Hold Your Baby," and "How Your Baby Takes Your Breast" (pp. 27-57) were meant to be read many times, paying attention to the details. The section entitled "Some Important Points" (p. 73) should be reread for review.

The mothers who used this book prior to publication found great success and did so by paying close attention to the details described in the text and demonstrated in the photographs. They reread parts of the book many times between feeds, and some moms reread the book between babies!

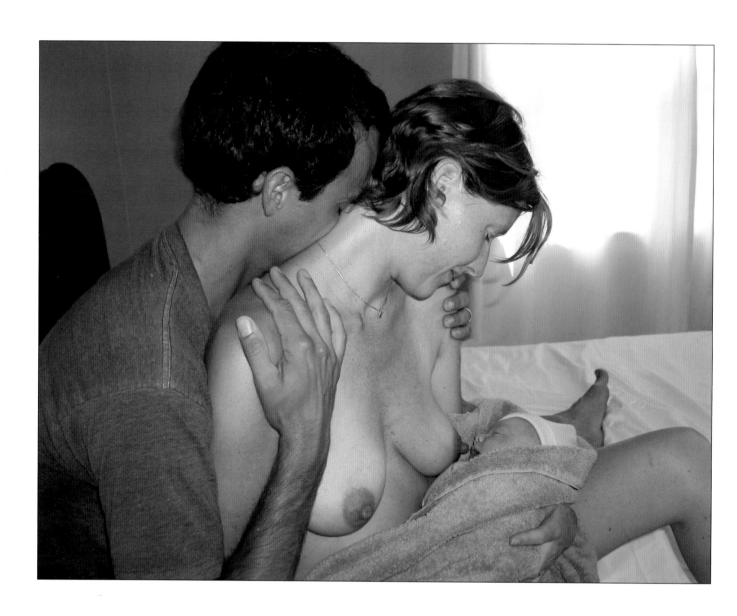

To experience the birth of a child
is to participate in the drama of creation.
Having experienced it
we will never be the same.

No child, no universe,
no mountain, sea or poem
was ever born without great labor,
yet when that labor's done
there exists a thing of beauty,
with a life all its own.

To experience the birth of a child
is to witness the promise of tomorrow.
Our hopes and dreams are all renewed
by the child who rests peacefully,
safe within our arms.

author unknown

On the day you were born...

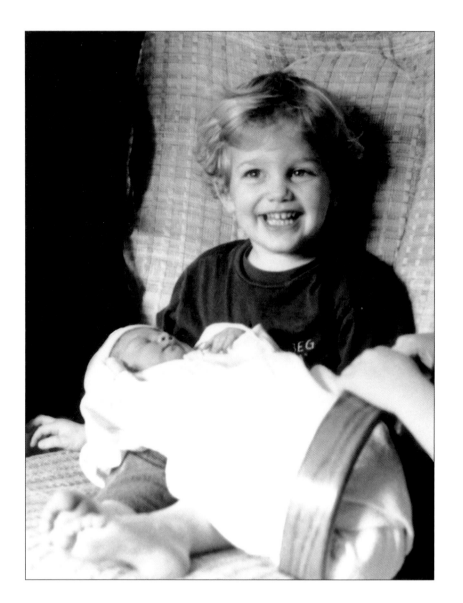

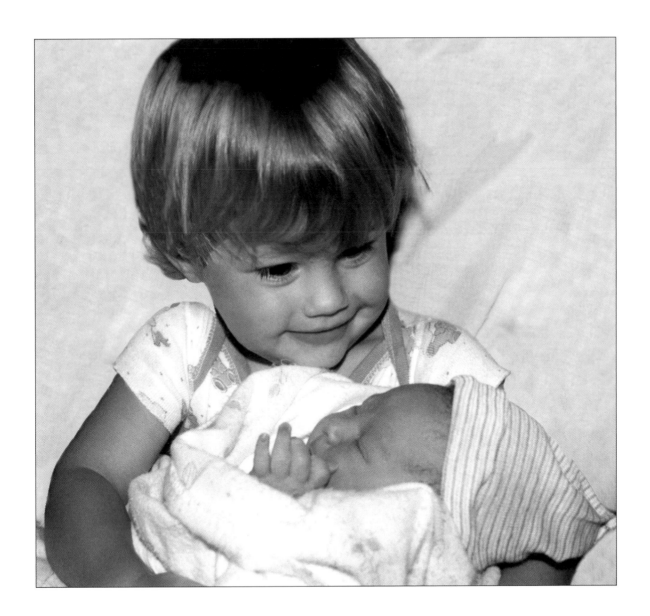

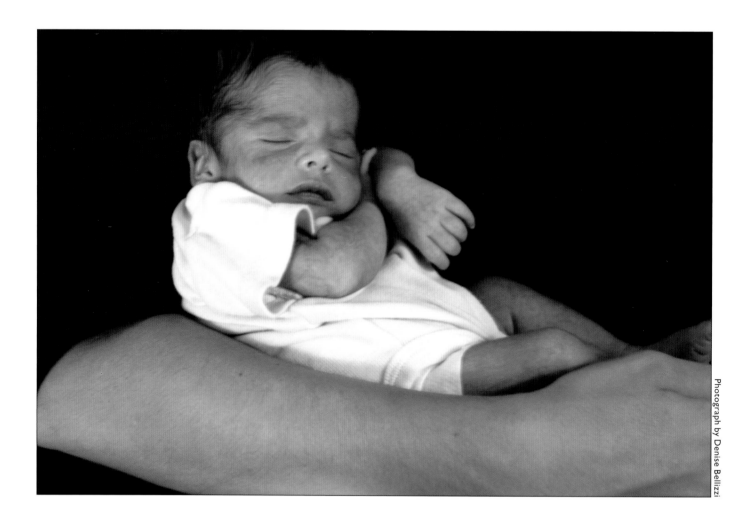

When I approach a child he inspires in me
two sentiments: tenderness for what he is,
and respect for what he may become.

Louis Pasteur

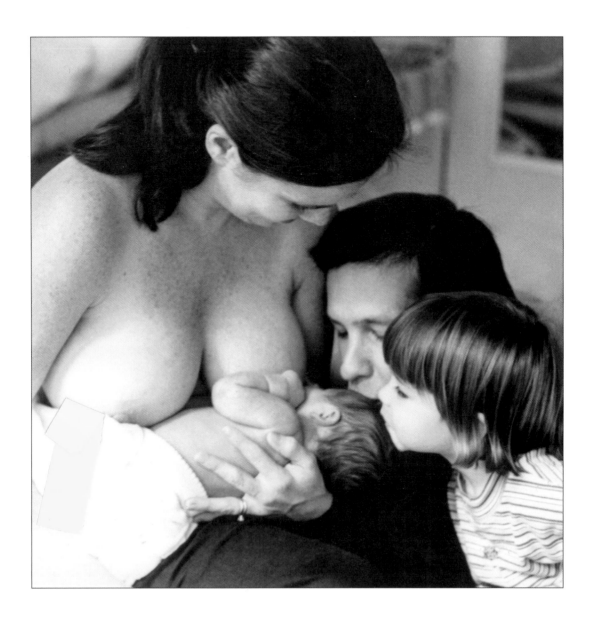

Sweet voice,
sweet lips,
soft hands,
and softer breasts.

John Keats

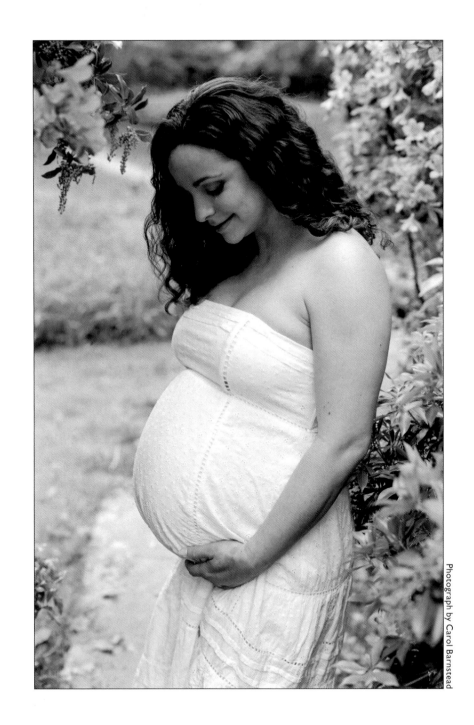

Introduction

You've picked up this book because of your interest in breast-feeding. Perhaps you are considering breastfeeding or already have your baby feeding from your breast. I have written this book to and for you, the mother, and your family, whether your baby is in your arms, your womb or your heart. Perhaps you are someone who wants to help a breastfeeding mom. This book can help you do that.

You may be somewhat apprehensive because of the stories you have heard from friends, family members and strangers about how difficult breastfeeding can be. Many mothers say they had to stop or give up. These stories can undermine your confidence in your body.

There are usually simple reasons for the problems mothers have encountered that lead to varying difficulties, such as sore nipples, babies fussy at the breast, sleepy babies, frequent feeds, babies not being satisfied, and colic. The purpose of this book is to emphasize certain key points that provide for an enjoyable breastfeeding experience for both mother and baby. A mother naturally wants a happy, contented baby during and after a feeding, and a satisfied baby can be a source of much pleasure and pride for the breastfeeding mom.

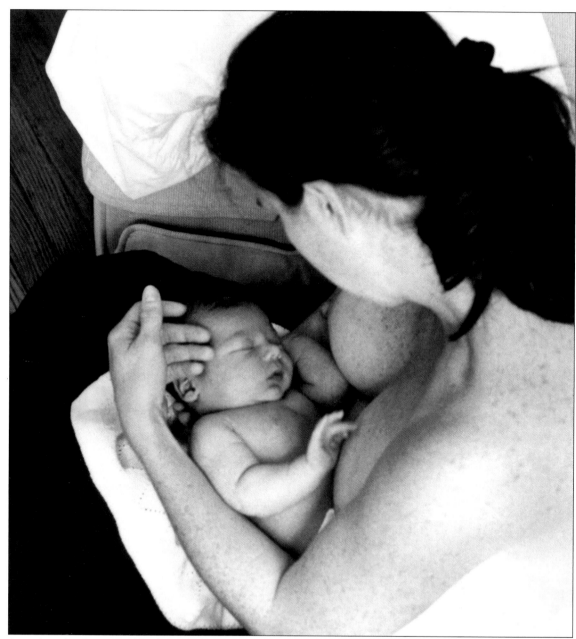

A newborn has been nourished entirely from his mother's body.

Gaze at your baby now, and realize that he has been nourished completely from your body since his life began, and nature provided your body with the ability and wisdom for this miracle to continue.

You will learn ways of holding your baby and bringing your baby to the breast that are imprinted early in life in women in other societies where breastfeeding is the norm. The steps are simple but may take a little time to learn because women automatically hold their babies and their breasts in ways that work for bottle-feeding since that is what most of us have imprinted in our minds. The details are important here, so don't be overwhelmed by them; just follow them step-by-step from the beginning, and read them over a few times before your next feed.

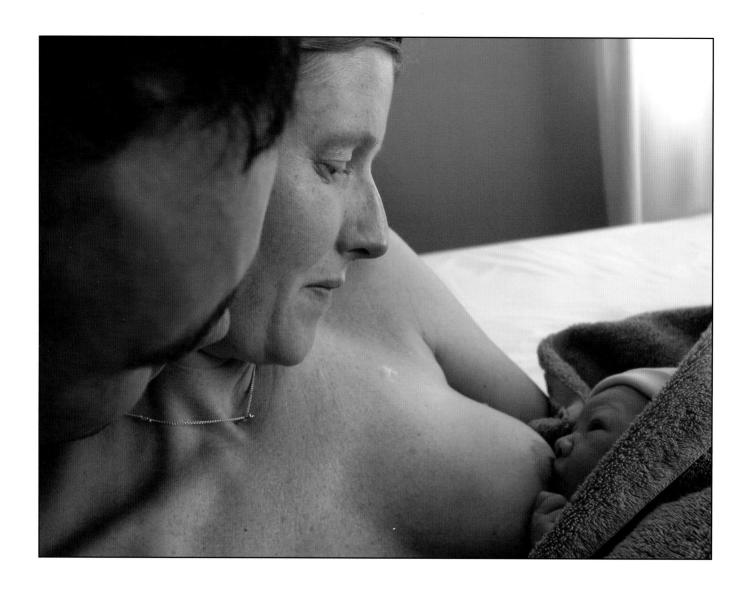

Feeding Your Baby for the First Time

If possible, and it usually is, give your baby the opportunity to breastfeed within the first hour of birth. You will have plenty of time to rest after that because your baby will take a very long nap. Sometimes you need to be proactive because, depending on where you have your baby, initiating breastfeeding may not be given enough attention, when there are so many distractions and routines to follow. With a Cesarean birth the baby can be brought to the mother's chest even as the incision is being closed.

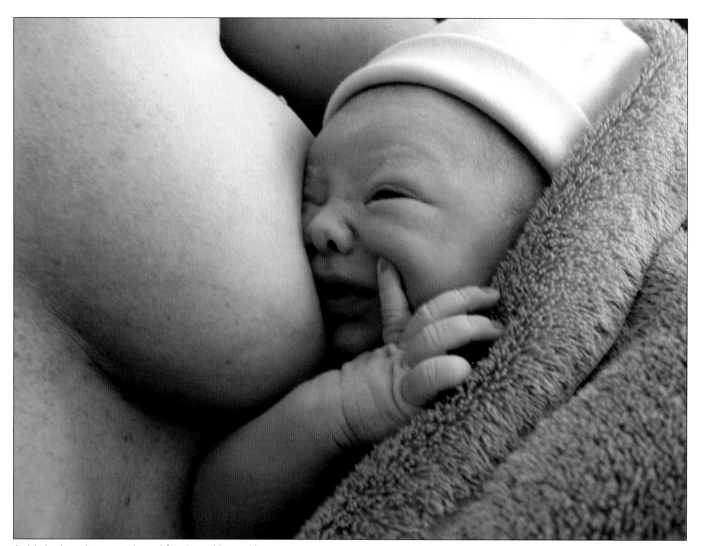

At birth, there is a mutual need for close skin-to-skin contact.

When there is no interference with babies and mothers post-partum, it becomes obvious that there is a mutual need for close skin-to-skin contact. Hold the baby close to you after the birth if you can, allowing her to nuzzle your breasts. She will try to feed if she is ready. Otherwise, just be with her until you have the quiet, calm time to focus on feeding your baby, if possible, within the first hour of the birth. Even if feeding must be delayed, it is still often possible to have periods of close physical contact that benefit you both.

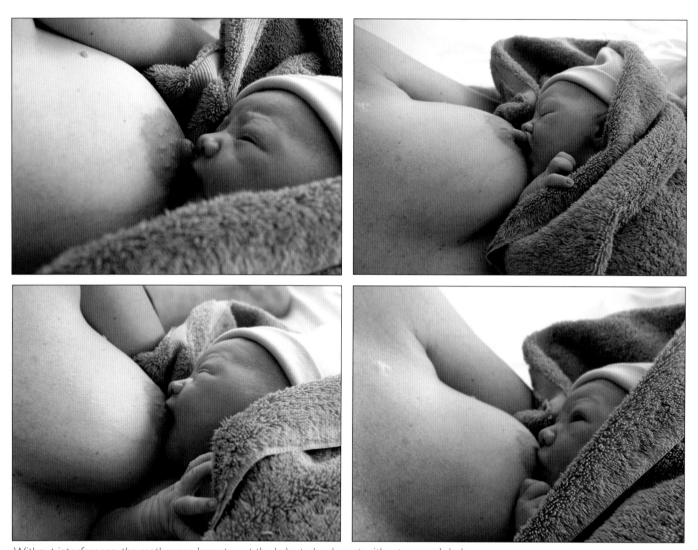

Without interference, the mother can learn to put the baby to her breast without anyone's help.

The first hour of life can be a wonderful window of opportunity. As Dr. Michel Odent, a French obstetrician and author of such books as *Birth Reborn* observes, "It has been my experience, in thirty years of obstetrics, that when a mother and her baby are allowed to be alone together in the first two hours after birth the mother will learn how to put the baby to her breast correctly, without anyone's help" (Arms 203). Newborn babies will actually crawl up to the breast and latch on if left without interference on the mother's abdomen at birth. Dr. Lennart Righard, a Swedish pediatrician, studied and filmed this phenomenon (Righard, *Delivery Self Attachment*).

A Note about Visitors

You may have to limit visitors and the time visitors spend with you in these early days, even when you are in the hospital. A good rule for visitors in the first week is to limit their stay to 15 minutes per visit. You should also request that they provide a meal. This may sound demanding to you, but it is unreasonable to expect a woman who has just given birth (some of whom are recovering from major abdominal surgery) to have enough energy for a continuous flow of company. At first, she does not notice how much energy this requires, energy that she needs to take care of herself and the baby. Limiting visitors will also help Dad. He needs to conserve his energy because he is going through a major transition, and at the same time, needs to be completely available to Mom and baby.

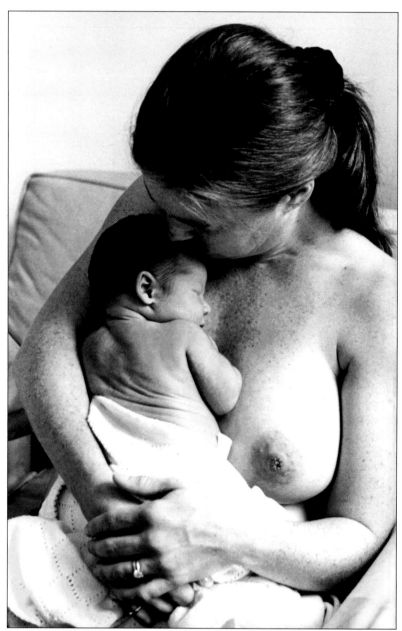

Skin-to-skin contact can calm your baby and ready her for feeding. Wrap a blanket around you both and snuggle.

The Importance of
Skin-to-Skin Contact

Undress your baby to her diaper, and undress yourself from the waist up. Snuggle your baby close, and cover you both with a blanket, allowing the warmth radiating from your body to keep your baby warm.

As you tune into the feelings this simple closeness creates, discover the calming effect it has on you and your baby. This skin-to-skin contact is especially important when feeding must be delayed.

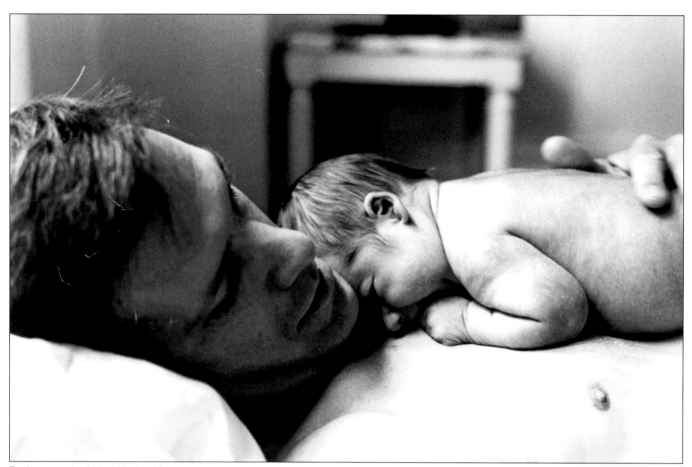

Dad can soothe baby skin-to-skin, too.

This closeness is therapeutic for both you and your baby, will increase your milk supply, and your baby will have a much easier time at the breast when it is time to feed her. It also can help when you are having difficulty getting your baby to take your breast. Allow time for this skin-to-skin contact throughout the day and night. This kind of skin-to-skin contact is good for dads and their babies too!

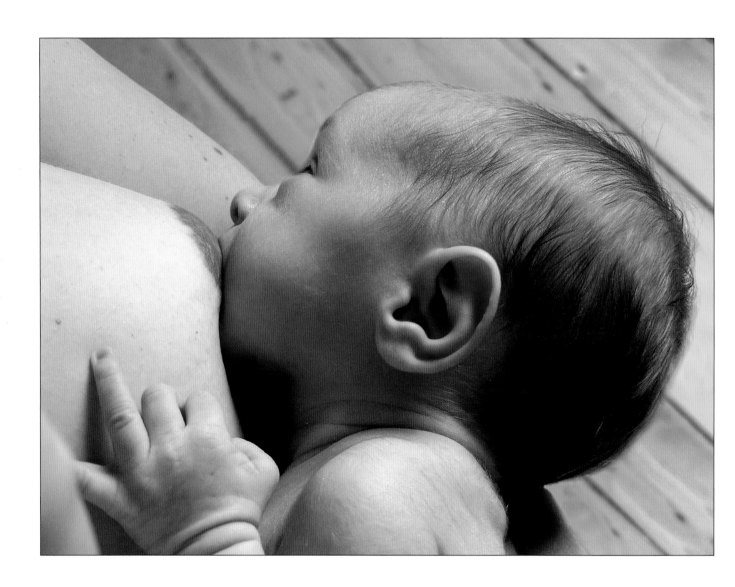

Studies have shown that mother/baby skin-to-skin contact keeps the baby as warm as an incubator and helps turn things around for those babies having difficulty with breastfeeding. The mother's ability to keep her baby warm cannot be disputed and is even more amazing when considering the premature baby who can have an especially difficult time maintaining a stable body temperature. The research of Dr. Ludington-Hoe reveals the synchronous ability of mothers, skin-to-skin with their premature babies, to unconsciously regulate their babies' skin temperatures in the correct range (Appendix A).

Dr. Ludington-Hoe's findings are not only fascinating, but are something every new mother and her medical providers should fully understand. This synchrony between mother and baby skin-to-skin has implications for helping any baby with difficulty, including breastfeeding problems.

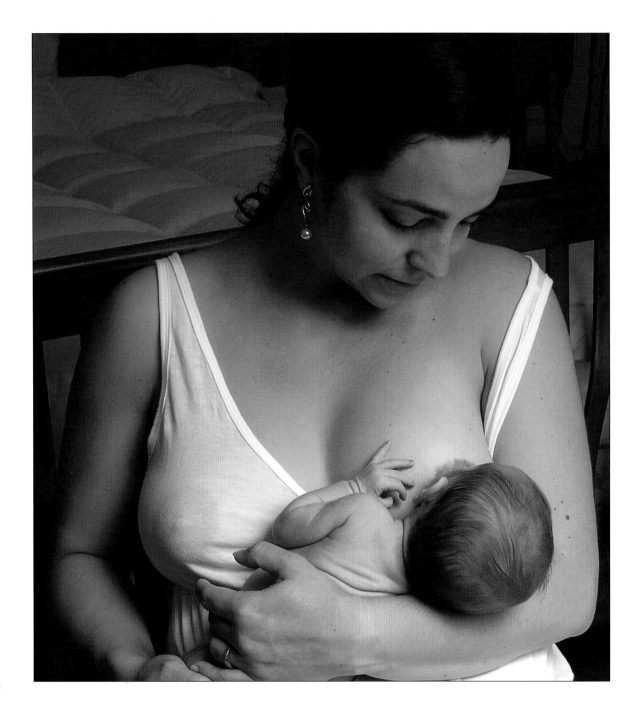

Positioning

Proper positioning from the very beginning prevents prob-lems and minimizes the effort required to breastfeed. Breast-feeding ease is dependent on your posture and comfort, and how you hold your baby so that he can get the breast in his mouth in the way nature intended for efficient and comfort-able suckling. PAIN IS NOT NORMAL. If feeding your baby hurts, you need to make some changes that will become clear as you continue to read. Take a few deep, calming breaths before you begin.

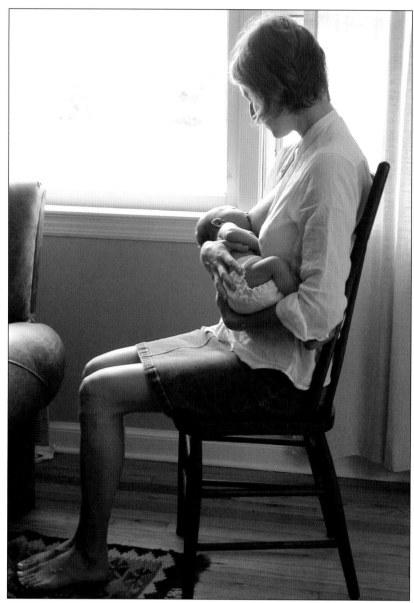

Mom's back is straight allowing the baby to latch properly. A footstool or phone book under her feet would allow her knees to be raised slightly above her hips making the baby more secure in Mom's lap. Pillows or rolled blankets under Mom's arms would provide additional support.

Posture

If you are sitting, you need to have your back straight, your lap almost flat and parallel with the floor, knees raised slightly above your hips, and your feet flat on the floor or footstool. You do not want to be leaning back because your breasts are then pulled away from your baby. Be careful not to be hunched forward because the baby cannot get enough of his mouth on the underside of the breast. Soft couches and chairs often force you to hunch forward, and your knees end up much higher than your hips, not giving your baby the space he needs.

Make yourself comfortable by supporting your body, arms and feet. You may use pillows, rolled towels or blankets for your arms and body. Thus your baby's weight is supported by the pillows, and you can easily respond to the baby's mouth opening and get the baby to the breast. A footstool or telephone book under your feet allows your knees to be slightly raised above your hips so you can feel your baby securely on your lap without the lap sloping down.

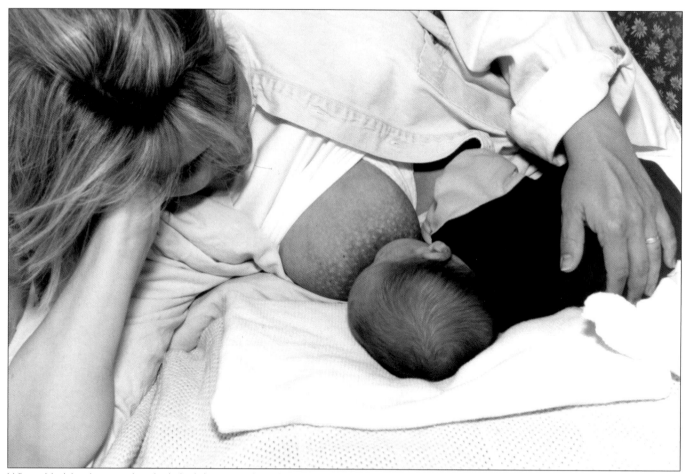

When side-lying, be sure that the baby is low enough so that he can take the breast from below.

You may want to lie on your side. It is helpful to have a pillow between your knees and a thin pillow under your side and breast so that the baby can come up to your lower breast from below. Also, you should place the baby closer to your feet than you expect so that the baby can get enough of his mouth on the underside of the breast. This placement is important because it allows the baby's tongue to have more contact with the areola than the roof of the mouth. The tongue milks the breast. Thus it should have greater contact with the areola than the roof of the mouth. The position of the baby's mouth is explained further in the section, "How Your Baby Takes Your Breast."

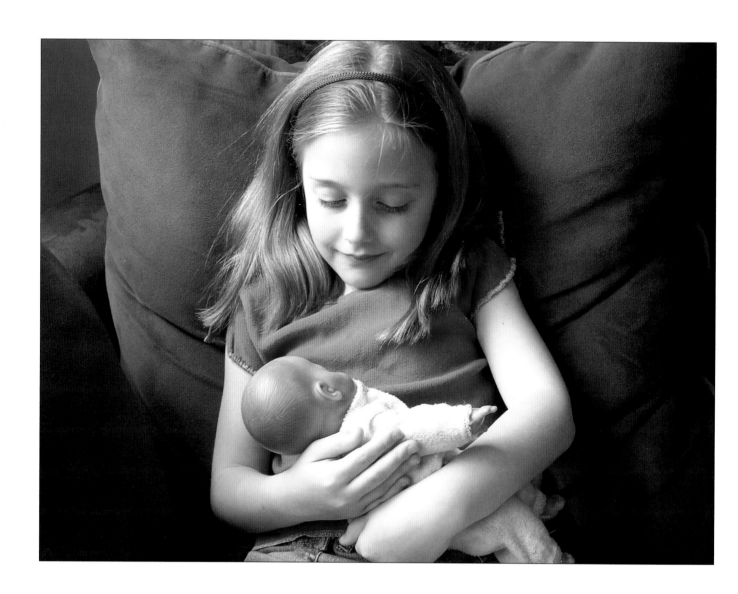

How You Hold Your Baby

Watch a small child cradle her doll when she is not giving it a bottle. She holds her doll so that she can look down and make eye contact with her baby. She doesn't have to look to the side as she does when she lifts the baby up and to the side to bottle-feed. This is because she naturally places the doll so the baby's head is near the center of her lap. Like the little girl holding her doll, when you breastfeed your baby, it is best if his head is more to the center of your body than you might expect.

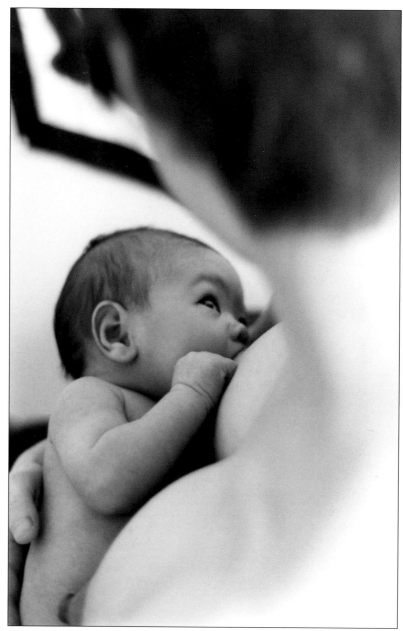

His body is facing your body but turned slightly away from yours so that his eyes can make contact with yours as you look down at him.

You may need to place a firm pillow or rolled blanket or towel in your lap to bring your baby close enough to your breast so that he can come up to the breast from below without straining. You should not have to lift your baby with your arms or lean forward. It is also important that your baby not be raised too high. You may need two different-sized supports at the baby's head and bottom because the baby's bottom is usually lower. Hold your baby, lying on his side, with his body snugly against your body. His body should be facing your body but turned slightly away from yours so that his eyes can make contact with yours as you look down at him.

The baby's head, neck and body should be in a straight line. He should be well supported, especially from his head to his bottom, with your arms and hands. Your arms and hands should then be resting comfortably on your pillows or rolled blankets. Make sure his bottom is snuggled in close to you. Often when you focus on the mouth and head, his bottom falls away from you some. As a result, the baby is less snuggled in against your body and may become fussy at the breast.

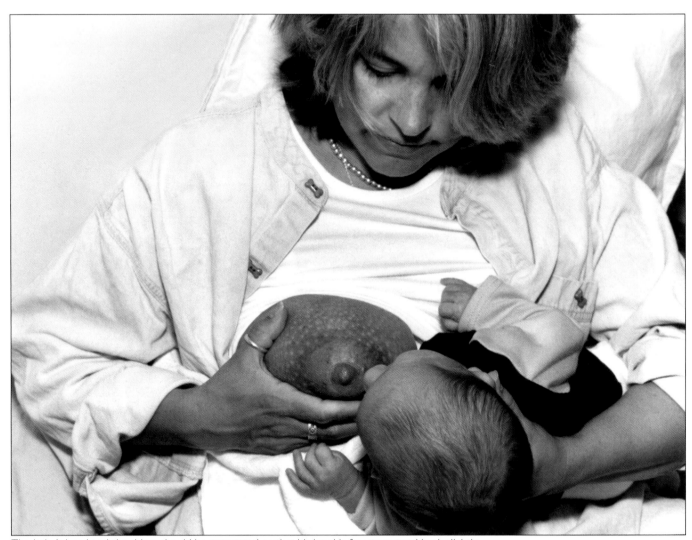

The baby's head and shoulders should be supported so that his head is free to extend back slightly.

The baby should be held just below your nipple as you get ready to bring him to the breast. His nose or upper lip, not the center of his mouth, should be in line with the nipple. The nipple will actually point to the baby's nose or upper lip. Be sure to wrap the baby's legs around your side enough to bring the baby's head more toward the center of your body than what you would do for bottle-feeding.

The baby's head and shoulders should be supported so that his head is free to extend back slightly and the chin reaches the breast first as he is brought to the breast. Be careful not to flex the baby's head, pressing his chin into his chest.

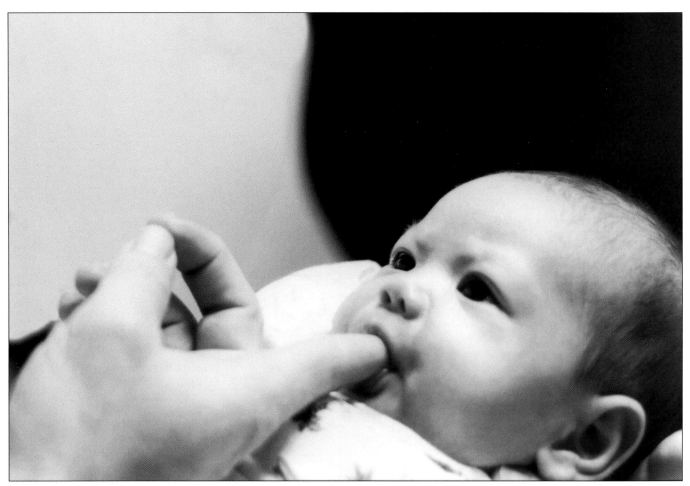

If the baby is getting fussy, try to calm him with skin-to-skin contact, snuggling him, or putting your finger in his mouth, fleshy side up allowing him to draw it in as he would the breast back into the arch of the roof of his mouth.

If his arms and hands are getting in the way, you may need to wrap the baby's arms at his side, or place the baby's hands on your breast as if he is holding the breast. If the baby is getting fussy, try to calm him with skin-to-skin contact, snuggling him, or putting your finger in his mouth, fleshy side up allowing him to draw it in as he would the breast back into the arch of the roof of his mouth. Stroke the roof of his mouth gently with your finger to entice him to suck. After he has calmed down, try to bring him to the breast.

You may need to support your breast as you bring the baby to the breast. Place your fingers under your breast and against your ribcage at the junction of your breast and ribs, and your thumb on top of the breast far back away from the areola. Do not squeeze the breast; support it. Some women find it helpful to support the breast with a scarf wrapped around the underside of the breast and tied in the back of the neck.

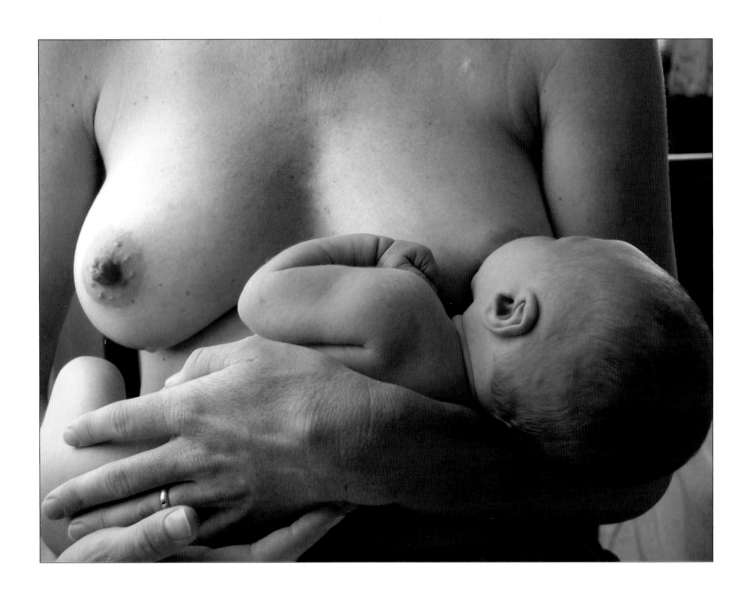

Now you are ready to bring the baby to the breast. DO NOT TWIST OR MOVE YOUR BODY OR YOUR BREAST TOWARD THE BABY. BRING THE BABY TO YOU, ALLOWING HIM TO TAKE YOUR BREAST. He is not given the breast in the same way a bottle is given to a baby.

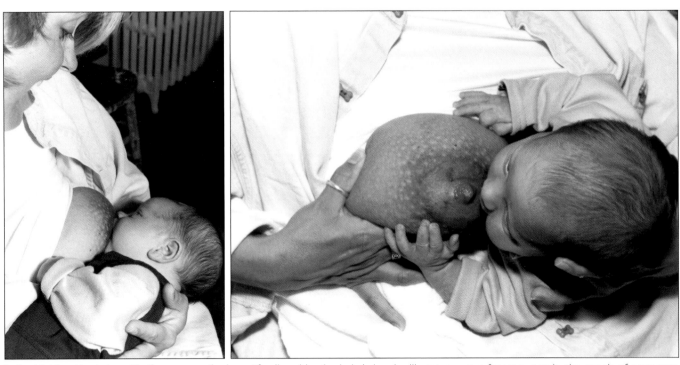

Left: Holding the baby with the arm on the breastfeeding side, the baby's head will rest on your forearm, not in the crook of your arm.
Right: If you use the opposite arm, you will place his shoulders in the palm of your hand with your fingers extending upward, supporting his head lightly. Your elbow or forearm of that arm will snuggle his bottom close to your body.

How Your Baby Takes Your Breast

Your baby is able to latch onto your breast best if his head and shoulders are supported so that the baby's head is free to extend back slightly as you bring the baby to the breast. You allow for this by the specific way you support the baby's head and shoulders. You can hold him either with the arm on the breastfeeding side or with the opposite arm. If you use the opposite arm, you will place his shoulders in the palm of your hand with your fingers extending upward, supporting his head lightly. You may find your fingers on the back of his head or on the side of his face or both. Your elbow or forearm (depending on the length of your arms) of that arm will snuggle his bottom close to your body, with his legs wrapped around your side and his back resting on the inside of your forearm.

If you use the arm on the breastfeeding side, you will support his neck, shoulders, and base of his head on the inside of your forearm, just below your elbow. Do not cradle him in the crook of your elbow as you would do for bottle-feeding.

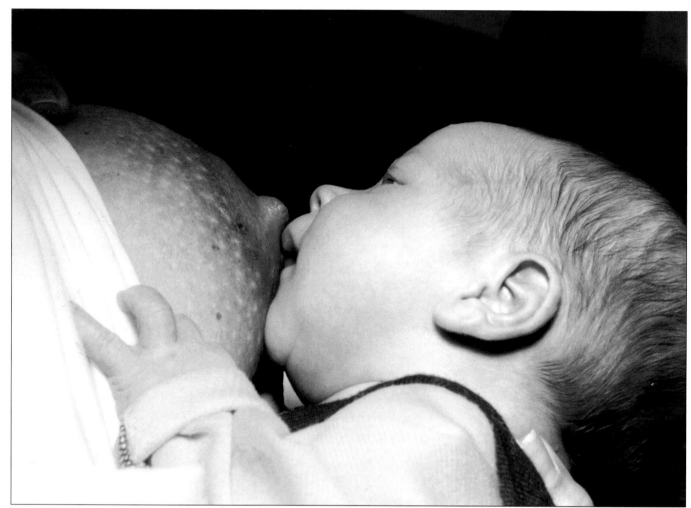

The nipple should point to the baby's nose. The chin should touch the breast first.

Before the baby's mouth is open, THE NIPPLE SHOULD POINT TO THE BABY'S NOSE, and the baby's mouth should be slightly below the breast. Bring the baby's mouth close enough to the breast to just tickle the areola lightly, the softer the touch the better. Wait for his mouth to open wide, and be patient. It could take a couple of minutes.

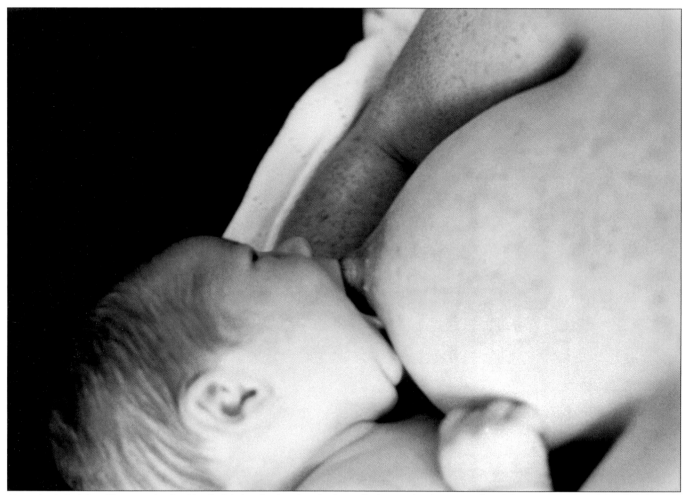

Here the baby's head is properly tilted back slightly, allowing the nipple to slip just under the upper lip, while the chin touches the breast.

As the mouth is opening, bring the baby quickly to the breast, with his head extended back slightly so that his chin and lower jaw touch the breast first. Aim the baby's bottom lip as far back on the areola and away from the nipple as possible, while the baby draws in the nipple and areola into his mouth. The nipple should slip just under the upper lip as the breast is drawn in. If the mouth doesn't open wide enough to reach the nipple, DO NOT PUSH YOUR BREAST INTO THE BABY'S MOUTH. Instead, adjust the baby's position before he opens his mouth again so that the nipple points to the upper lip instead of the nose, and try again. When the baby is latched on correctly, he will have more of the areola with his lower jaw and tongue than his upper jaw. This may be difficult to see. What you will see is that your baby will be snuggled in close to the breast with his mouth open wide, his chin pressing into the breast, and his nose just off the breast.

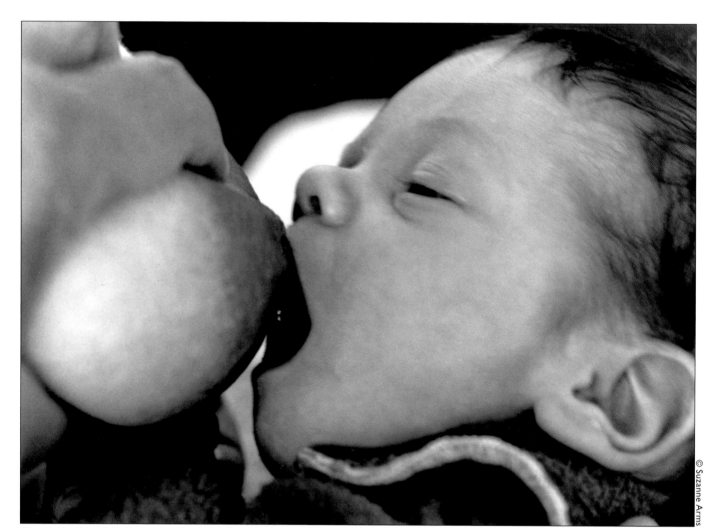

The nipple should slip just under the upper lip as the breast is drawn in.

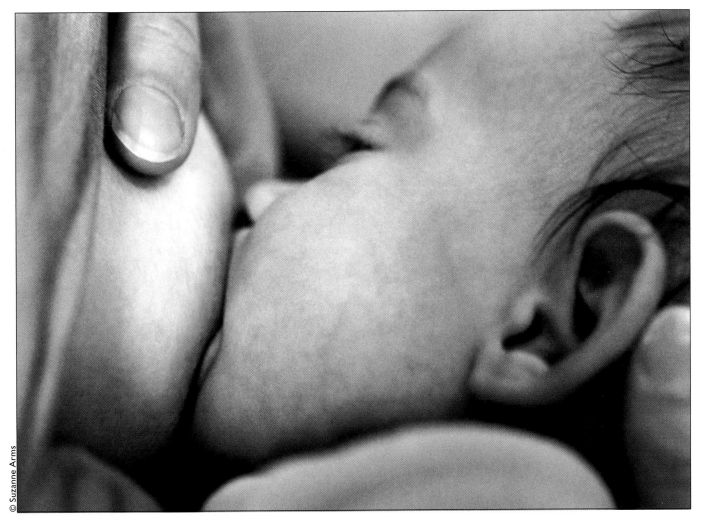

Chin pressing into the breast, nose just off the breast.

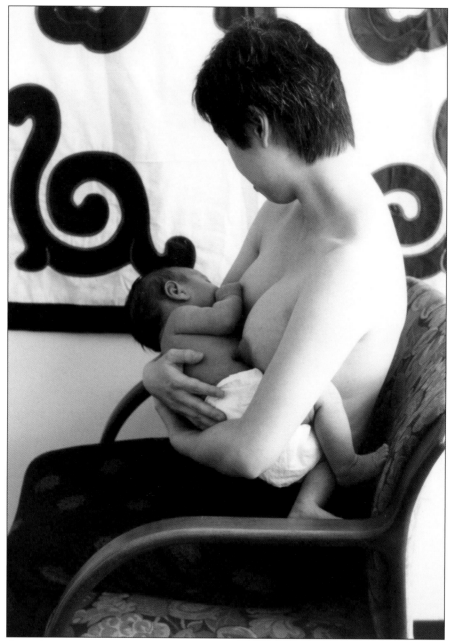

Once the baby is latched on well, you can adjust your arms to cradle your baby comfortably.

When the baby takes the breast in this way, the nipple is drawn to the back of the mouth (at the junction of the hard and soft palate) where there is no friction. You can visualize this as the nipple pointing to the roof of the baby's mouth where it is suspended freely in the arch without any friction. You should therefore experience no pain as the baby nurses.

The tongue draws in the breast and compresses it to draw milk. The upper jaw is passive. The tongue can draw in as much as possible and has maximum contact with the areola when you aim the bottom lip as far back on the areola as possible. The result is the tongue is positioned so that it can express the milk most efficiently.

Once the baby is latched on well, you can adjust your arms to cradle your baby comfortably.

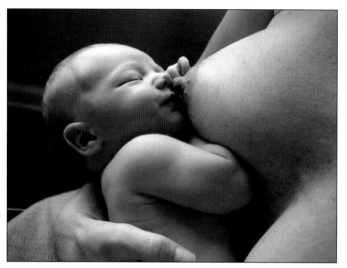

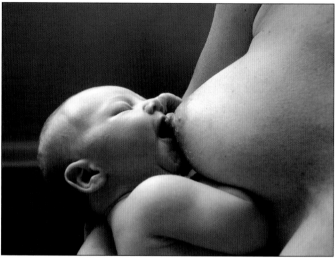

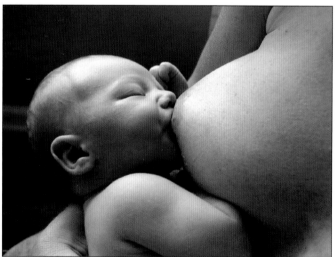

In the first picture, a six-day-old baby is seen content at the mother's breast in a good position to take the breast. He is seen yawning in the second picture but still in good position and then seen in the final picture latched on well. He is the same baby seen latching on well just after his birth on p. 18. The proper positioning and latch are already well-establlshed for both Mom and baby.

Opposite page: Here we see a one-month-old who takes the breast and latches on well. When his mom is readying him to feed, she brings him to the breast so that his lips touch the areola as lightly as possible. As the baby latches on, the chin hits the breast first. His mom learned these techniques when her baby was a newborn, and they are well imprinted on both baby and Mom. Note the mouth position, relative to the nipple/areola.

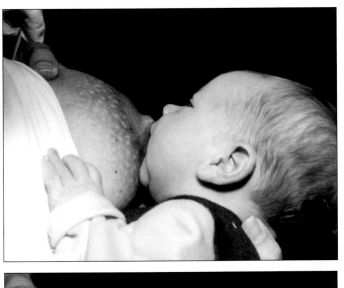

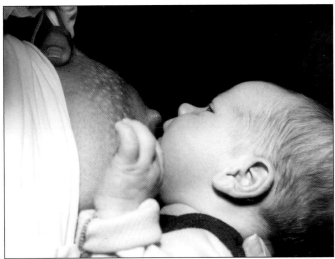

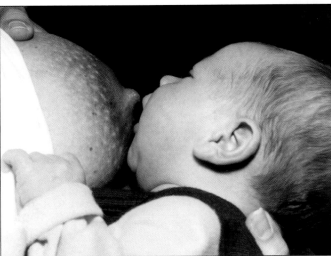

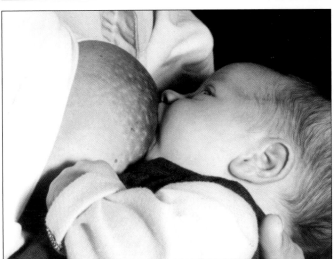

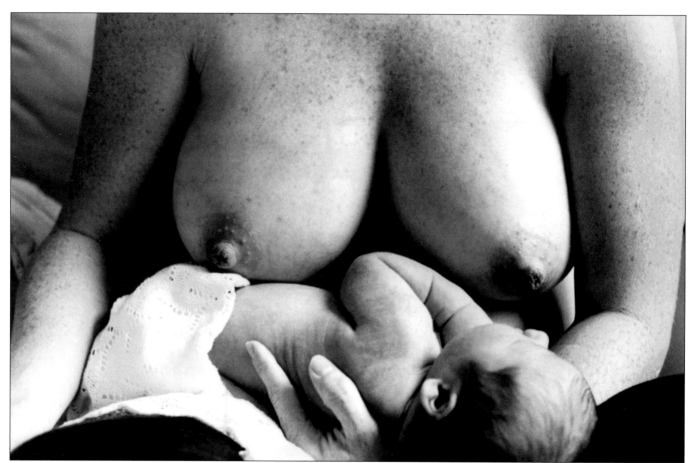

Most women's nipples naturally point outwards.

It is interesting to note that when most women look down at their unclothed breasts, the nipples point outward, instead of straight ahead. We unconsciously push our breasts to the center of our bodies to make our nipples point straight ahead as they do in bras. We don't want to push our breasts in this way when we breastfeed.

The natural position of the nipple pointing outward allows for the nipple to point to the roof of the baby's mouth when bringing the baby to the breast. Indeed, nature has an ingenious design to ensure painless, efficient feeding at the breast, when holding the baby in a way that is not affected by bottle-feeding imprinting.

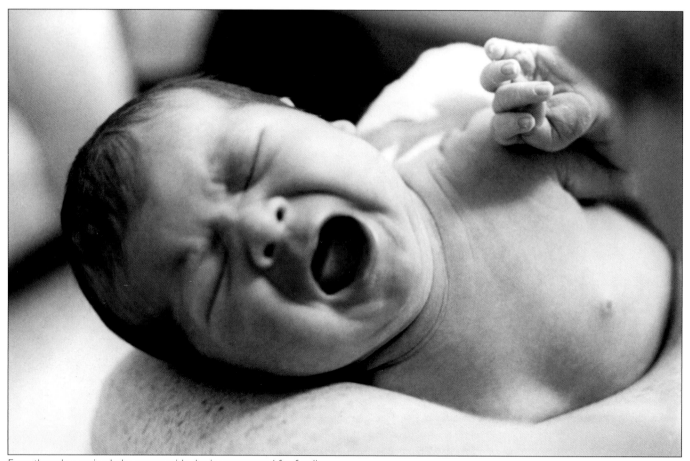

Even though a crying baby opens wide, he is unprepared for feeding.

A Note about Crying

Even though the baby's mouth opens wide during crying, do not bring the baby to the breast. His tongue is
back when he is crying, and he can't latch onto the breast
correctly, as he does when you elicit the reflex opening
of his mouth, where his tongue comes forward over his
lower gums.

If you experience pain after your baby has latched on and is
feeding, take your baby off your breast gently, first by slipping
a finger in the corner of his mouth between his gums to break
suction and then taking him off the breast. Then try again.
You may want to take a few deep, calming breaths. Then
comfort him and try again.

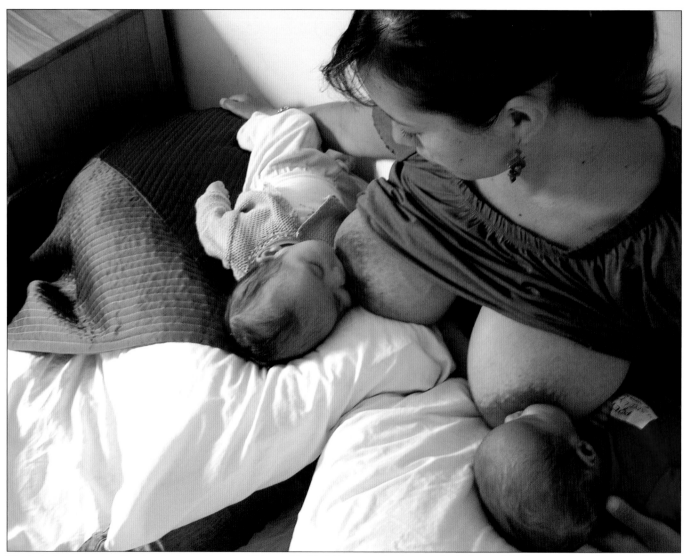

The baby has grown so that her feet would push off the wall behind Mom, moving her too far in front of the breast. Mom placed the baby so that the baby's legs were angled away from Mom's body, allowing the baby's head to be positioned properly. Additional pillows placed behind Mom would have provided more leg room while allowing the baby's body to be up against Mom.

More on Positioning and Holding Your Baby for a Good Latch – the "Football Hold"

Sometimes early on, mothers prefer the "football hold." The goal is the same. That is, you want the nipple to end up back in the arch of the roof of the baby's mouth, and you want maximum contact of the tongue with the areola for pain-free efficient milking of the breast. To achieve this goal, the baby will be further back toward the back of your seat than you expect, bringing her head back far enough and underneath the breast so that the baby does not come up and over the breast. If the baby's feet push off the back of your seat, you may need to allow for more room for the feet as demonstrated in the picture on the previous page. You will need one or more pillows to support your arm that is holding the baby. You want the baby to be high enough to reach the breast but low enough to have room to latch from the underside of the breast.

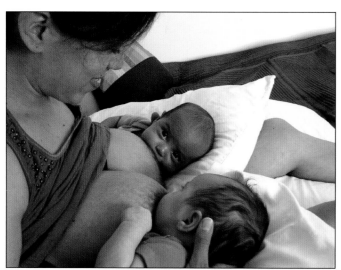

Mom's fingers are on the back of the baby's head for support.

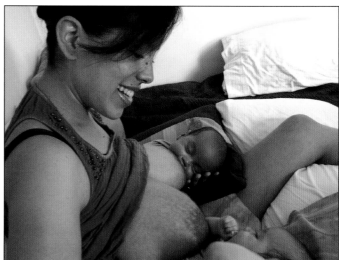

Mom's fingers are on the side of the baby's face for support.

You support the baby's head and shoulders with your fore-arm and hand similarly to the way you hold the baby when the supporting arm is opposite the breastfeeding side (as discussed and photographed on pp. 42-43).

On the preceding page, the mother is nursing her twins using the "football hold." Notice the different placement of the supporting hand on the far twin in the first and second pictures. Both pictures show proper support of the baby's head where Mom's fingers extend up from the palm of her hand that is supporting the baby's shoulders.

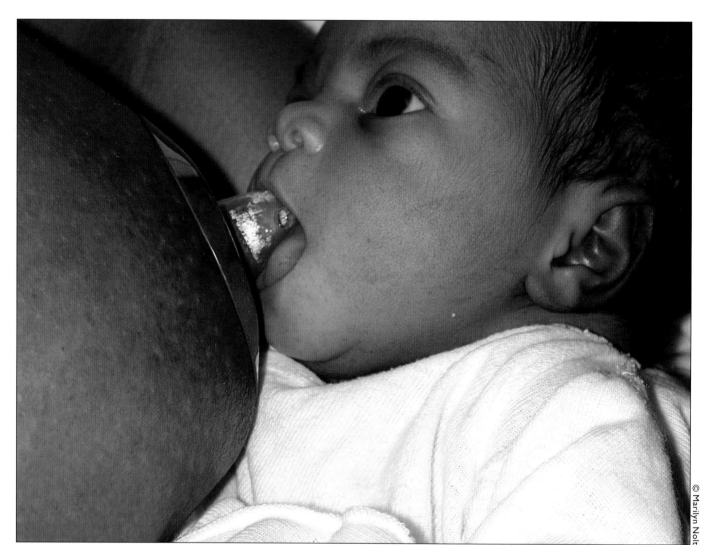

When a baby does not latch onto the breast, the nipple shield can be used temporarily after the milk "comes in."

© Marilyn Nolt

Is Your Baby 'Refusing' Your Breast?

A baby who does not latch on to your breast, despite your efforts, may appear to be too restless, too sleepy or uninterested. This is usually temporary. Spend prolonged periods of time with your baby skin-to-skin, allowing spontaneous opportunities for breastfeeding. If possible, spend 2-3 days in bed with your baby allowing others to take over the household duties and to feed and care for you.

Uninterrupted periods of physical contact between you and your baby can settle your baby into breastfeeding. Refer to "The Importance of Skin-to-Skin Contact" (p. 21). If your baby remains restless at the breast despite skin-to-skin contact, wrap your baby prior to feeding. If your baby seems to be too sleepy for feeding, look for the feeding cues described on p. 83 prior to feeding, and attempt to waken your baby using the techniques on pp. 85-89.

Nipple shields, as shown on the previous page, are often given to women when their babies are not latching on. It is important to note that they should not be used before the milk "comes in." They should be used only temporarily while you and your baby are learning the proper position and latch. Prolonged use of the nipple shield can cause a decrease in milk supply. Attempt to feed your baby without the shield at each feeding, so that you don't lose the opportunity for the baby to latch onto the breast when he is ready (usually within 24-48 hours).

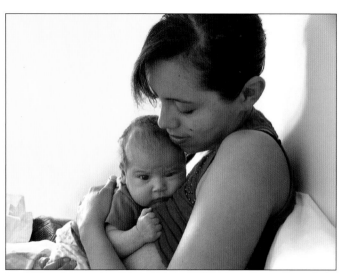

Some snuggle time with Mommy calms a fussy baby.

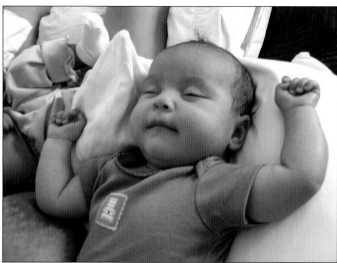

After some calming time, she was able to complete a satisfying feed.

In my experience, I rarely recommend the nipple shield because proper position and latch allows the baby to feed from the breast with ease. If a baby can nurse with a shield, he can be at the breast in a few days with proper attention to the latch. Usually the problem is not getting the breast in the mouth far enough and/or not waiting for the baby's reflex opening of the mouth before bringing the baby to the breast.

The "nipple portion" of the nipple shield easily fills with milk with compression of the breast by the baby's mouth and/or your hands. It provides a reservoir of milk that is easy for the baby to extract. The ease of extraction helps when babies are not extracting milk well from the breasts as often occurs with premature babies, but it also happens with term babies who need a few days to attain proper position and latch. The difficulty is usually temporary, and the nipple shield is used during this transition.

If your baby is not feeding from your breast, pump your breasts and feed your baby the expressed milk until your baby is able to breastfeed. If you don't have a high-quality pump, you can hand express the milk. Pumping or expressing milk is important when the baby is not feeding at the breast. It is important not to be discouraged if you get little milk the first couple of days pumping. This is not an indicator of a low milk supply. Often it takes practice to elicit a letdown of milk, and in the case of hand expression, to learn the technique that works for you. You can encourage a letdown by smelling or seeing your baby, gently massaging your breast, and gently stimulating the nipple with light touch.

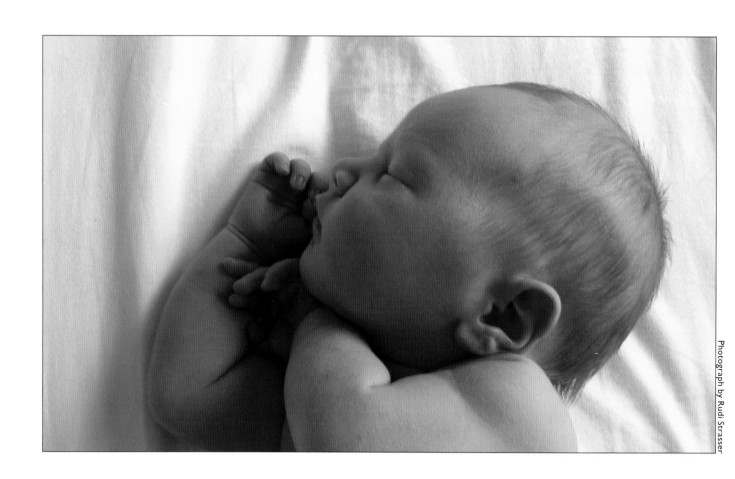

66

Hand Expression of Milk

There are many ways of hand expressing milk, and every mother can make adjustments to this basic technique to suit her body. After encouraging the milk to let down, place your thumb on the upper edge of your areola, and cup your hand under your breast with your forefinger directly below your thumb and your lower three fingers against your ribs. Your milk is coming from deep within your breast and you want to gently push the milk along, as well as squeeze the milk out of the ducts that lie just below the nipple and areola. You do this by gently compressing your breast between your thumb and forefinger. At the same time, you push your hand back toward your ribs, and then gently roll your thumb and forefinger forward. Be careful not to slide your hand and fingers over your skin, as it can cause irritation. Adjust your hand position as needed to continue the milk flow.

Your milk may drip or spray from your breast. Collection is possible with a bowl-shaped or wide-mouthed container under the flow of milk. However, collection and pumping are usually much easier using a high-quality electric double pump.

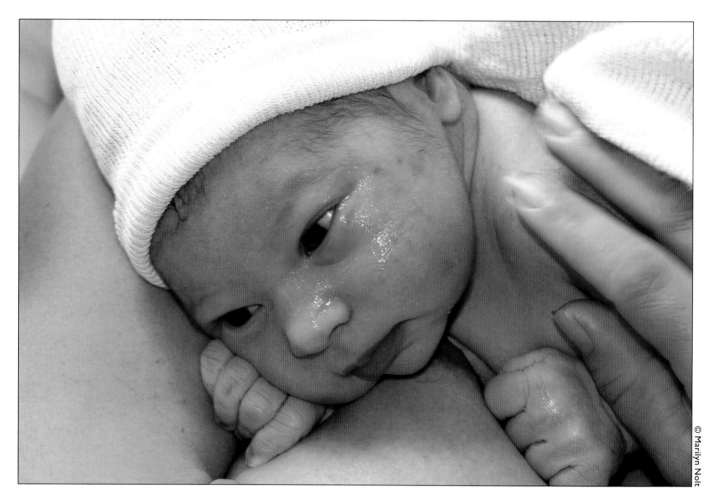

When this newborn is ready, he will respond to his suckling instincts.

Feeding Your Baby Expressed Breastmilk

If your baby is not feeding at your breast for some or all of his feeds, you can feed him expressed breastmilk from a bottle. The baby can transition from bottle to breast with proper attention to the position and latch. It is important that during the period with the baby off the breast, you pump or hand express regularly to maintain your milk supply, ideally pumping for most feeds that are not at the breast.

Pumping should not be painful and prolonged. If your pump is hurting you, don't use it. An adjustment to the vacuum setting or flange attachment size may eliminate the pain. Pumping should take no more than 10 to 15 minutes, and you should pump until the flow of milk stops. You can wait a moment after the flow stops to assess whether or not you get another letdown and then continue. Otherwise stop pumping. Early on, many mothers get very little volume. It is true in the early days with the calorie-rich colostrum and true even after the milk comes in, when moms don't easily experience a letdown with the pump. The volume usually increases with time, and you should continue pumping regularly, despite the small volume, until you can feed your baby at the breast. Low volume obtained during pumping does not mean you have a low milk supply.

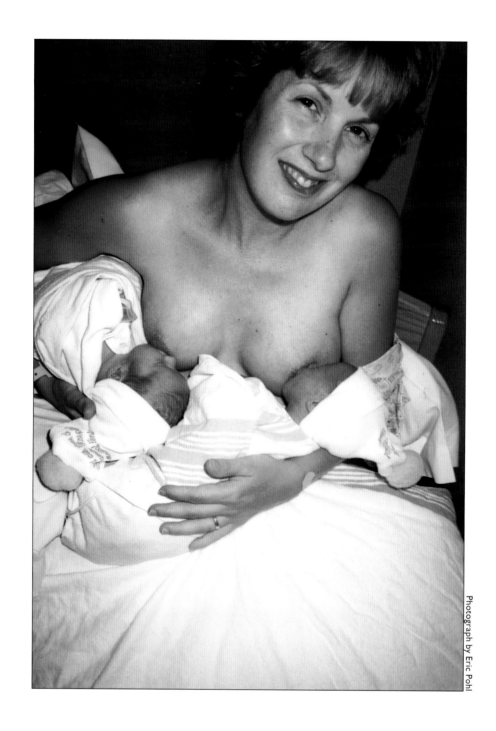

Photograph by Eric Pohl

In my experience, I do not see "nipple confusion" since babies return to the breast after weeks on a bottle. Chloe Fisher and Sally Inch note in their letter to the Editor in *The Journal of Pediatrics* entitled, "Nipple confusion— who is confused?" that a baby will go from bottle to breast when he is calmed and helped to attach to the breast correctly and gently (Fisher). Chloe Fisher, a midwife, has been helping mothers with breastfeeding since 1956 and because of her success, has been helping colleagues, including midwives and doctors at their request, since the 1960s. Sally Inch began working with breastfeeding mothers as a midwife in 1976 and as a specialist in breastfeeding since 1993. Their combined experience gives much credibility to their statement that babies do not refuse the breast secondary to being bottle-fed.

It is helpful when feeding the baby from a bottle to tickle the baby's lips with the nipple and allow time for the reflex opening of his mouth, followed by allowing the baby to draw the bottle nipple into his mouth. When a baby is accustomed to opening his mouth wide and drawing the nipple in to feed, the transition to the breast can be easier.

Appendix E provides information about other methods of feeding expressed breastmilk.

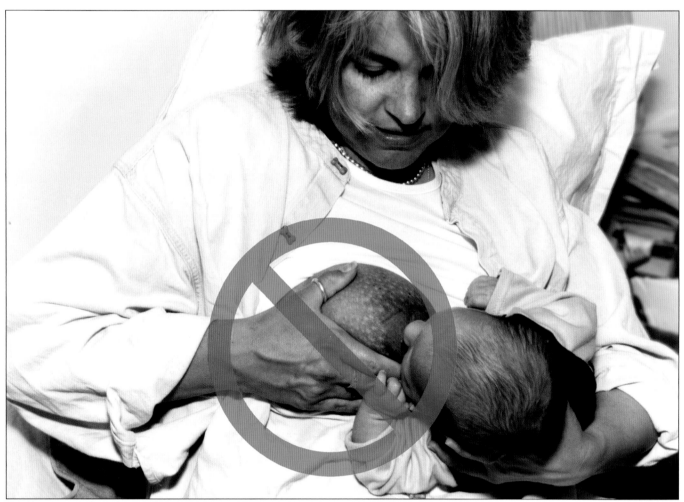

Don't move your breast toward the center.

Some Important Points

Make sure you bring your baby to the breast quickly enough as he is opening his mouth wide. Otherwise, his mouth may have already closed some by the time he gets to the breast. THE BABY COMES TO YOU, NOT THE BREAST TO THE BABY. When you push the breast to the baby, you disrupt the relative position of the baby's mouth to the breast.

Make sure the baby is tucked in close enough so that his chin is right up against the breast, and his nose is just slightly off the breast, allowing him to breathe. His nose should not be buried into the breast, and you should not need to pull your breast away from the baby's nose to let him breathe.

When you bring the baby to your breast after checking that your positioning is correct, make sure you do not move your breast at the last second during latching, in an attempt to center the nipple in the baby's mouth. You do not want the nipple centered. This last-second movement of the breast is one of the hardest things to get women to stop doing because of bottle-feeding imprinting. If the nipple is centered, the lower jaw and tongue cannot extract the milk as efficiently, and you may become sore. Remember, you want the nipple pointing to the roof of the baby's mouth and the lower jaw and tongue to take more of the areola than the upper jaw.

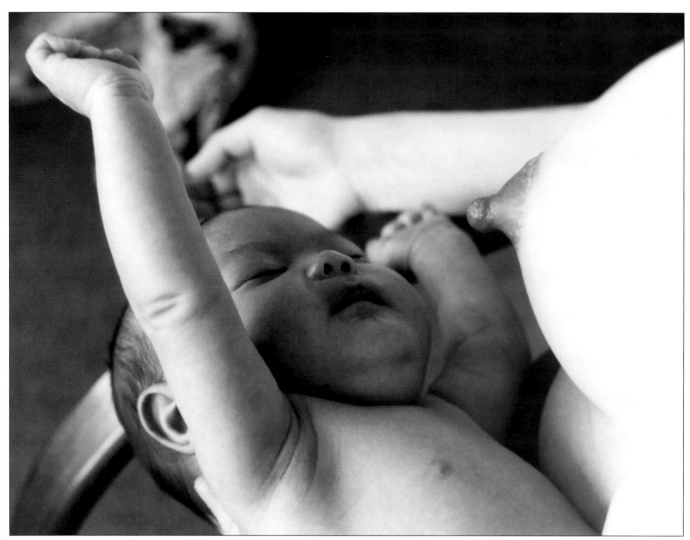

Sometimes it's easy to tell when your baby has had enough.

Signs of a Good Feed

- Your baby is relaxed and snuggled in close.
- You don't experience pain.
- Your baby begins to suck strongly and rhythmically as she settles into the feed.
- Newborns have pauses between each bout of sucking a few times.
- The strength of the baby's sucks varies throughout the feed, but she does not suck rapidly and lightly.
- The pauses may lengthen throughout the feed, but she continues feeding until she comes off spontaneously.
- Your baby's suckling is characteristic of drinking. Your baby is taking in good amounts of milk when her mouth opens widely and pauses slightly before she closes it.

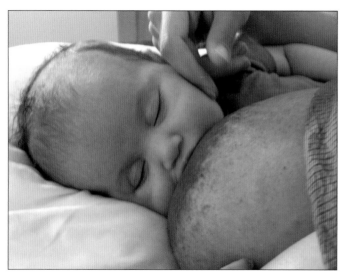 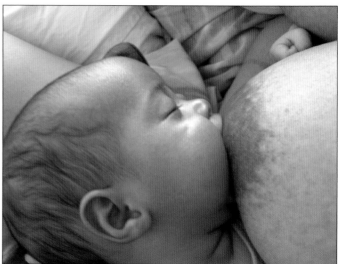

These babies are nursing well as they sleep. They are pausing between suckles here, but they had several minutes of the drinking type of suckle and continued in this manner after the pictures were taken.

You can see this characteristic movement of the baby's mouth if you watch her chin. Open-pause-close is one suckle; this pause is not the pause between suckles. The pause signifies a mouthful of milk. You may hear a quiet ''eh'' sound as she is drinking, signifying swallowing. But she may not make a sound loud enough for you to hear. Usually the baby's suckle will alternate between this type of suckle and nibbling suckles throughout the feed. If the baby has several minutes of open-pause-close type of suckles, she is having a good feed. If she nibbles only with light sucking, or has the drinking type of suckle for very little time, she is not feeding well (Newman, *Is My Baby Getting Enough?*).

Take the baby off the breast if she seems distressed, or you are not experiencing the signs of a good feed. Take a few calming breaths and comfort her. You may want to take some time to be skin-to-skin with her for a few moments before trying again. Try again, remembering your posture and how to hold your baby, noting the relative position of her mouth to your breast as discussed earlier.

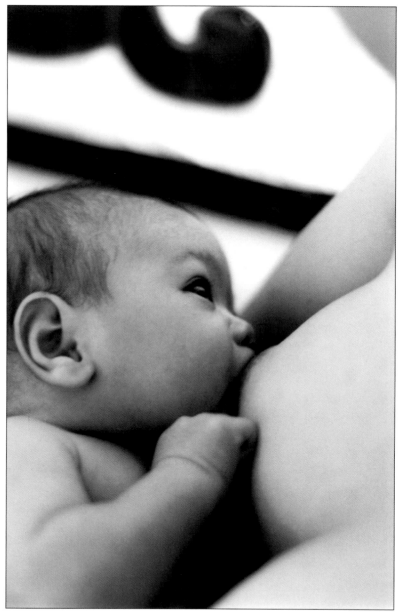

Be sure you allow the baby to stay on long enough to get the calorie-rich hindmilk. This baby's position allows him to gaze into his mother's eyes as he feeds from her breast for as long as he needs.

Insuring Your Baby Gets the Calorie-Rich Hindmilk

Feed your baby as long as he is suckling strongly on one side, and allow him to come off spontaneously. He gets more of the calorie-rich hindmilk the longer he feeds on one side because it is what the baby gets after he has taken the foremilk, which is higher in sugar and lower in fat. Getting enough hindmilk is very important to insure happy, satisfied babies, so don't take the baby off the breast before he is finished. Your baby knows how long he needs to feed to get the correct balance of foremilk and hindmilk. Good positioning allows the baby to suckle efficiently enough to get the hindmilk. The amount of time it takes to get the hindmilk is unique to each baby and may vary from feed to feed. Offer the second breast after you have burped him and changed him, if necessary. He may take only one breast at a feeding.

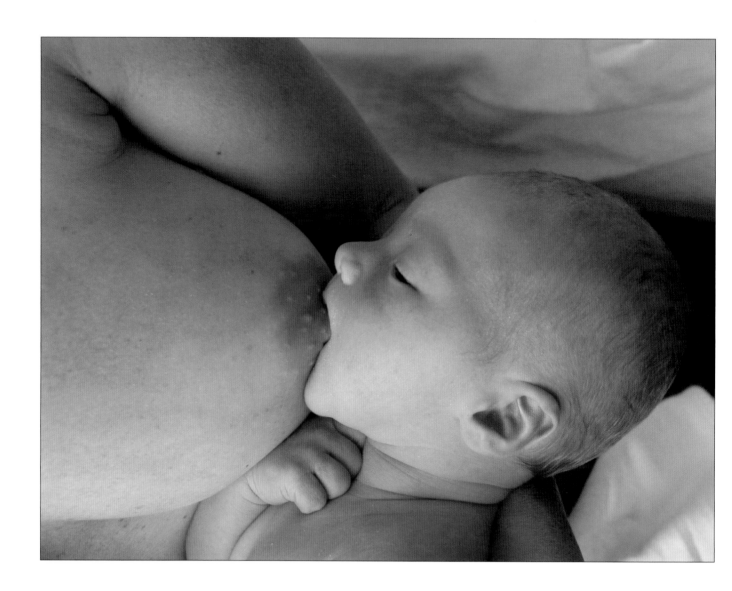

When to Review Your Technique

- Your nipples or breasts are sore.*
- Your baby has very long or frequent feeds.**
- Your baby is restless at the breast or shows no interest.***
- Your baby does not come off the breast spontaneously.
- Your baby does not seem satisfied after feeding.

* A good treatment for sore nipples is breastmilk applied to the nipple/areola and allowed to air dry. Sometimes sore breasts and nipples are not secondary to technique, especially if soreness occurs after a period of pain-free nursing. The most common cause in these cases is breast candida. It is very important to have this condition diagnosed correctly and not confused with mastitis secondary to a bacterial infection. Incorrect diagnosis and treatment can worsen the problem. Refer to the section on breast candida later in this book (p. 115).

**This observation is subjective. If the feed feels too long and too frequent, you probably can improve the situation. A guideline for a two-week-old baby feeding too long and too frequently would be: hour long feeds, more often than every two hours from beginning of feed to beginning of feed. If this happens sporadically during the day, it may be okay. If your baby is consistently feeding this way, check your technique.

***The importance of spending time skin-to-skin with your baby cannot be emphasized enough here. Refer to sections: "The Importance of Skin-to-Skin Contact" (p. 21), "Is Your Baby 'Refusing' Your Breast?" (p. 63) and Appendix A (p. 127) for both an explanation and rationale for this practice, and for methods to settle your baby into a good feed.

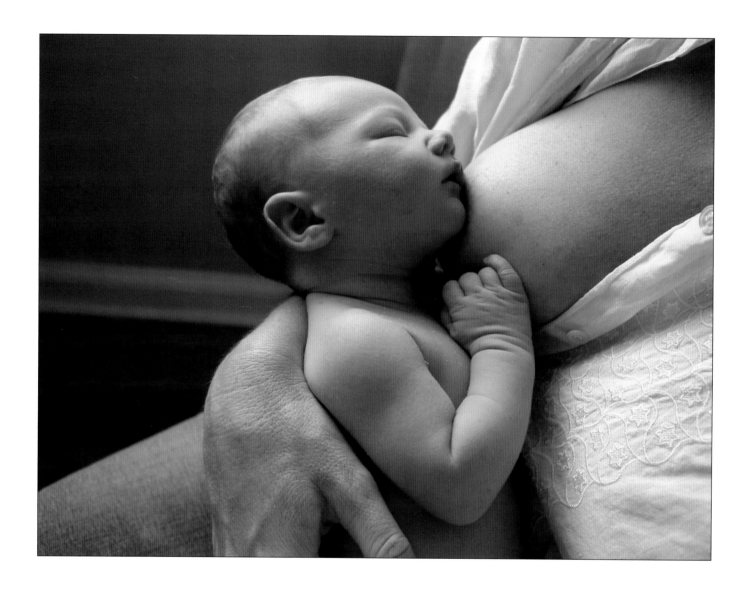

Do You Have a Sleepy Baby?

If your baby falls asleep at the breast shortly after beginning to feed, or does not wake to feed every 2-3 hours after the first 2 days, you may need some help with getting your baby awake to feed well.

The following are your baby's signals that he may be ready to feed. Note: crying is a late sign of hunger, so watch and listen for these signals first.

- Body movements, small sounds, hand to mouth movements
- Sucking on hand, arm or wrist or any sucking movements of the mouth and tongue
- Arms bent, hands fisted, hands at the face and head
- Open mouth, rooting, tongue out, mouthing motions
- Head bobbing around when being held
- Rapid eye movements under the eyelids

Your baby is in a lighter sleep state with any of these signs and is more likely to breastfeed well than at a scheduled feeding time of 2 hours when he may be in a deep sleep. After the first 24 hours of life, look for these signs every $1^{1/2}$ to 3 hours from the beginning of the last feed. Feed your baby about 8-10 times each 24 hours after the first 2 days of life. After some time (1-3 weeks of life) your baby will be waking to feed on his own, and you won't need to respond to these movements.

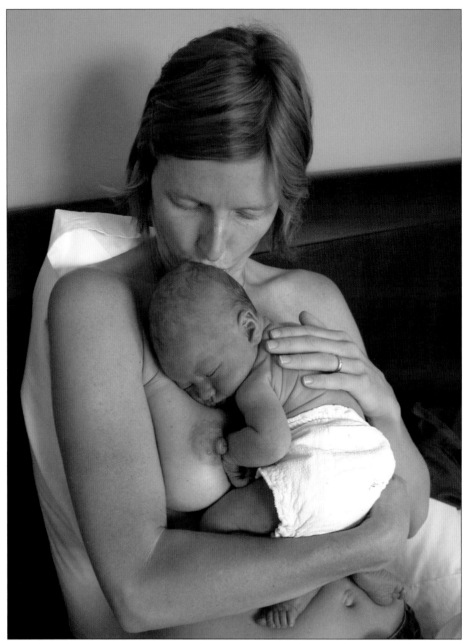

You may need to awaken your sleepy baby to feed.

How to Get Your Baby Alert Enough to Feed

After you see the feeding cues, you can waken your baby a little more by using the techniques below.

- Provide skin-to-skin contact as described earlier.
- Gently touch and stroke your baby all over: his face, his palms and soles, his body.
- Sit him up facing you.
- Gently rock him forward and backward and sideways.
- Slowly lift him up above you and bring him back down to your lap.
- Bring his hand to his mouth.
- Talk to your baby.

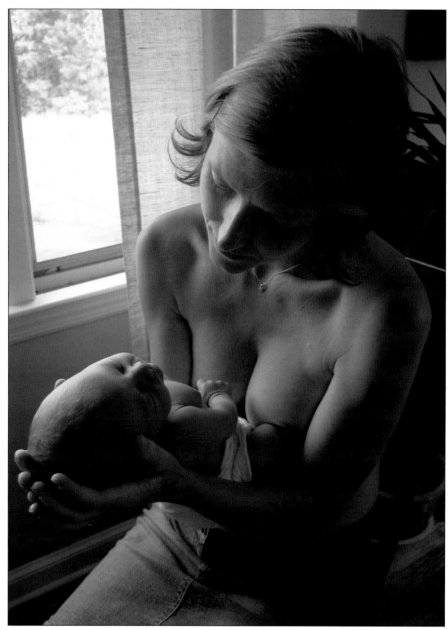

Skin-to-skin contact, touching, lifting, rocking and talking to your baby will help get him alert enough to feed.

You may want to express a few drops of milk onto your nipple and areola so that when you bring your baby to the breast, he can wet his lips or lick your breast just before he feeds.

If he falls asleep or begins to suck lightly shortly after he latches on to your breast, or before you think he may be finished with his feed, try getting him to suck strongly again by increasing the flow of your milk. You do this by placing your thumb on the top of your breast, your fingers on the underside of your breast, back away from the areola. Rhythmically compress and release the breast between your thumb and fingers, not so hard to cause discomfort, and stay back far enough from the areola not to change its shape.

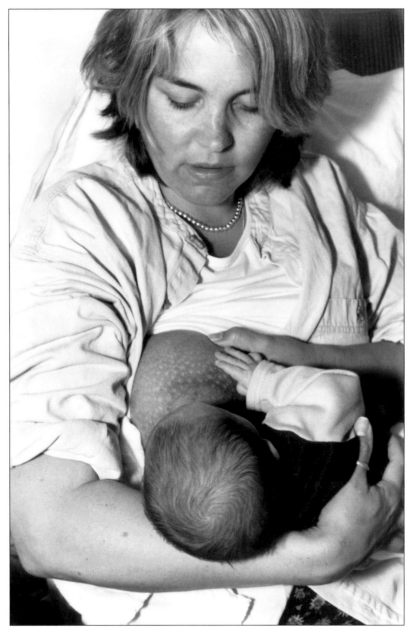

Breast compression: thumb above, fingers below, keep a consistent pressure while the baby sucks.

Try this a couple of times until the baby starts to suck again. When the baby starts to suck again, just hold the compression. Keep the pressure on your breast until the baby stops sucking. Then release the pressure and pause, to see if the baby starts sucking again without the compression. If the baby is no longer sucking, compress the breast again and repeat the process until the baby no longer sucks even with the compression. Wait a moment before taking him off the breast to see if you get a letdown that will start the baby sucking again. If he stops sucking and swallowing, take him off the breast. You can then offer the other side, perhaps after you burp him, if necessary.

The reason breast compression helps in the early weeks is because young babies often fall asleep at the breast when the flow of milk is slow. Older babies may pull away from the breast when the milk flow slows. Breast compression increases the rate of milk flow when it is slow, making it easier for the baby to extract the milk. Thus, the baby will not fall asleep secondary to a slowing of milk flow. The baby will get more hindmilk because he is encouraged to stay on the breast longer than he would have, giving him the chance to extract the hindmilk that comes later in the feed. Hindmilk is high in fat, allowing for a more satisfied baby.

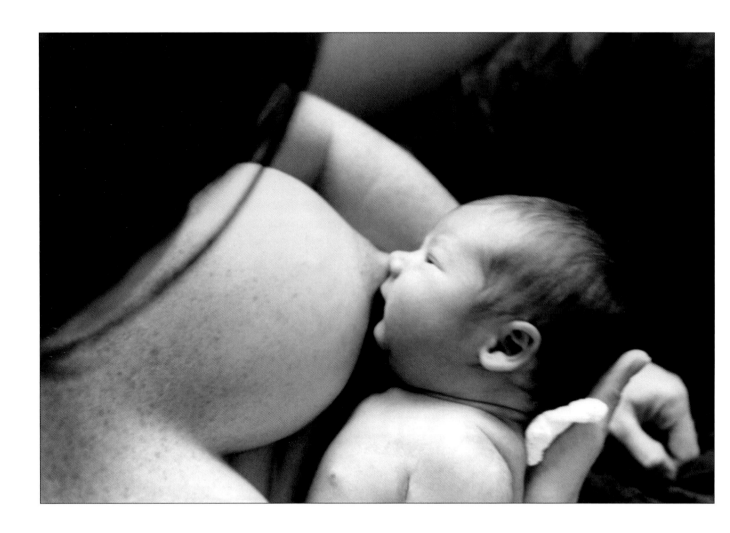

A Note about Wrapping Your Baby

Wrapping is often blamed for creating a sleepy baby. However, wrapping has so many benefits for the newborn in easing her transition from the womb, with its well-defined physical boundaries, to the expansive outside world. Her nervous system is very undeveloped, and you want to protect her from over-stimulation. Wrapping is excellent for her neurological health, and it keeps her boundaries intact. Just look for the feeding cues, unwrap her, and use the waking techniques just described. Then your arms and body become her boundaries as you snuggle her in close to feed her.

How Often Should My Baby Feed?

Ideally the baby will get a good feed within an hour of birth and then sleep for up to 8 hours. Expect to get 3 good feeds the first 24 hours and 6 good feeds the second 24 hours. However, you may bring the baby to the breast more often than this, attempting to nurse every $1^{1/2}$ to 3 hours from beginning of feed to the beginning of the next feed. These frequent attempts allow both of you time to practice the first couple of days. The baby does not need large volumes the first days while she is getting your calorie-rich colostrum. After the first 48 hours, you should expect to feed 8-10 times per 24 hours, in the early weeks.

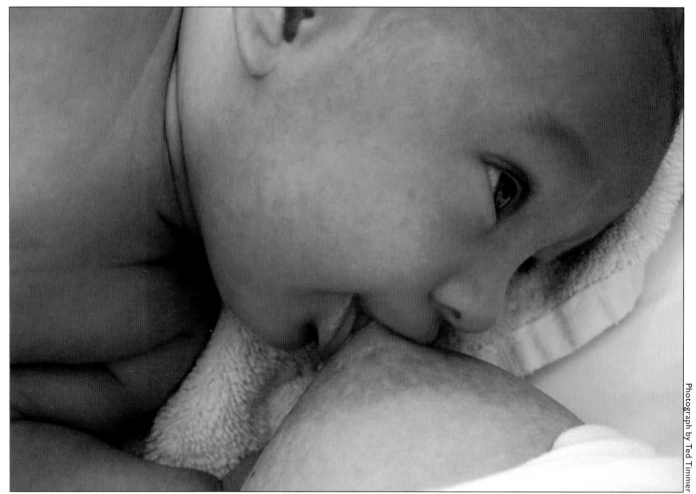

During a feed, a baby may pause to check in with Mom.

You should not limit the length or frequency of feedings at the breast. A baby who is feeding well will not be on the breast for hours at a time. If she is, she may not be latched on well and not getting the milk that is available to her. Also in the early hours and days, feeds take more time because you both are learning and the flow is slower. Allow yourself the time you need to get things started right. Using clocks to impose strict rules about length and frequency of feeding interferes with Mom's good sense about what her baby needs. Every baby is different. The first few days of life are very unpredictable. It is important to learn how to know if your baby has had a good feed; the clock then becomes irrelevant.

It is best for you and your baby to room in together if the baby does not need to be separated from you for medical reasons. You then can hear your baby's feeding cues before she is crying and too agitated to feed. This closeness allows you to snuggle her and have skin-to-skin contact whenever you wish, which is good for both of you physiologically. It provides for a good milk supply and a baby who is better able to feed. You can be easily misled by well-meaning caregivers who tell you that you need time away from your baby to rest. Rest near your baby, if possible. You can be the one to determine if you need time apart. Having early, frequent contact with your baby will make your life easier in the long run. You may find you rest better when you can hear, see, feel and smell your baby whenever you need to. After all, you were together for nine months. It makes sense to continue to be together if you do not desire to be apart.

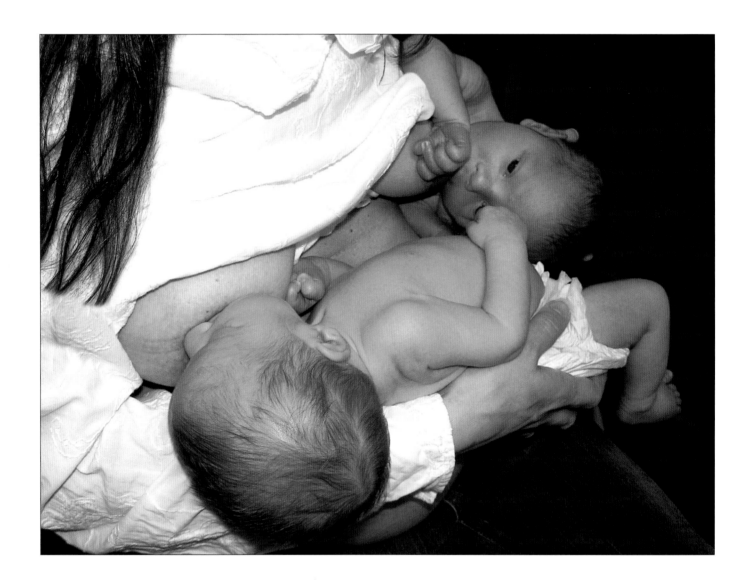

Avoid artificial nipples such as bottles and pacifiers in the early weeks until breastfeeding is well-established. Your baby will then take the breast as well as possible, and your milk supply will be stimulated the way nature intended, with the baby at your breast.

However, in my experience, babies do return to the breast after being placed on a bottle when attention is placed on proper position and latch. In my practice, the first time I see a baby is often after they have been in the hospital. Babies are placed on the bottle for a variety of reasons, including but not limited to, hospital routine, premature birth, and medical problems requiring placement of the baby in the neonatal intensive care unit (NICU). When the bottle is unnecessary, it is preferable to exclusively feed the baby at the breast. However, when the bottle is deemed medically necessary, I am confident that the baby will return to the breast when the bottle is no longer prescribed.

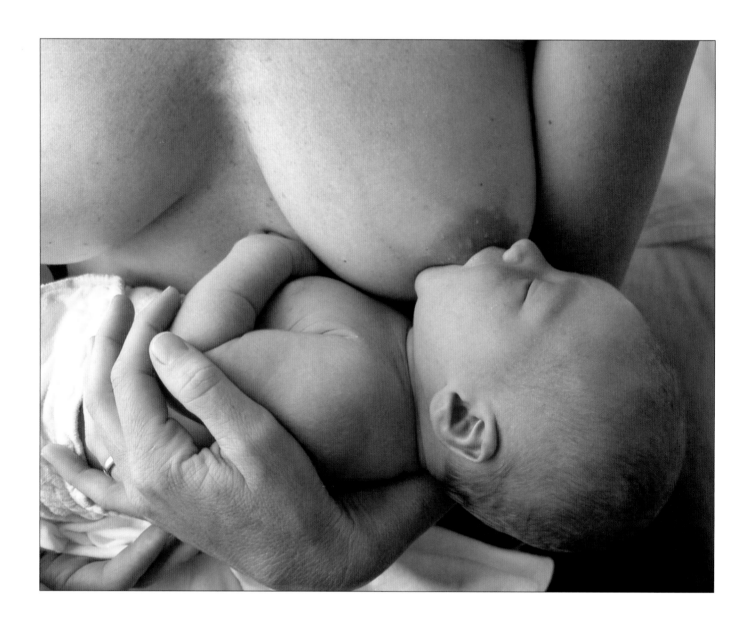

How Do I Know My Baby
Is Getting Enough?

The baby is showing signs of a good feed discussed earlier.

Baby's bowel movements are an indicator that the baby is getting enough calories in the early weeks. Meconium accumulates in the baby's intestines in utero. It is tarry and black or dark green and is passed during the first few days. By the third day the stools get lighter. They go from meconium to tarry and brown, to green, and by the fifth day are usually yellow and pasty or loose. There may be variations such as green or orange bowel movements. They may contain curds or mucus or have the consistency of shaving lotion. This variation does not indicate a problem. An exclusively breastfed baby whose bowel movements become lighter in color by day 3 is doing well (Newman, *Is My Baby Getting Enough?*).

Baby's urination is an indicator that the baby is getting enough fluid. With the disposable diapers it may be difficult to tell if the baby has wet her diaper. Place a dry tissue in the diaper at each change to check wetness.

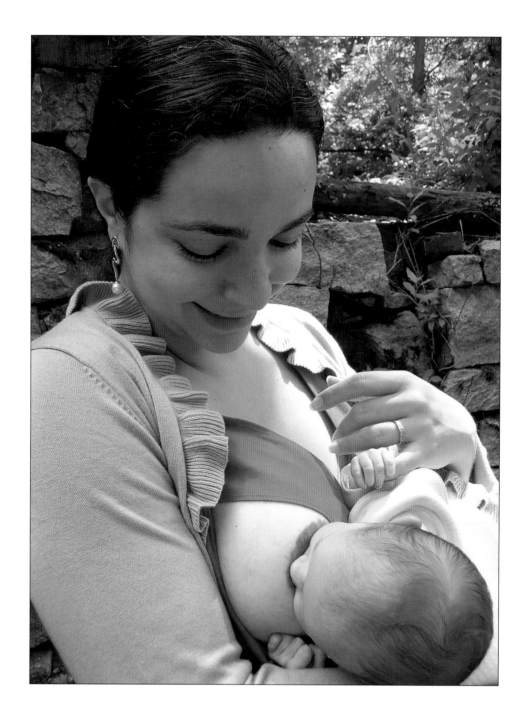

Counting Diapers – an approximation of what to expect:

Age in days	# wet in 24 hr.	# soiled in 24 hr.
1	2	1
2	3	2
3	3-4	3-4*
4	4-5	3 or more
5	4-5	3 or more
6	6-8	3 or more
7	8	3 or more

* many babies don't have this many the 3rd day and are fine - watch for lightening of the color

By the end of the first week, you should see a minimum of two substantial bowel movements per day. There is cause for concern if a baby under 3 weeks of age but older than 5 days does not have at least one substantial bowel movement in a 24 hour period. If this happens, you should have your baby checked by his health care provider.

Your baby may have a bowel movement with every feed. This pattern is normal. At around 3-4 weeks of age, the stool pattern may change from many stools daily to one daily or one every 3-7 days. As long as the baby is well and comfortable, and the stool is pasty or soft, it is not a problem. It is normal.

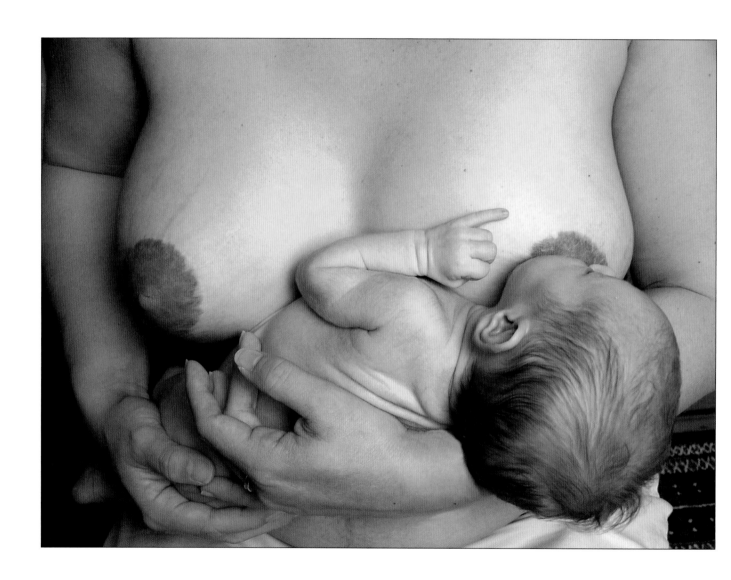

Dealing with Engorgement
(Painful, Swollen Breasts)

Engorgement often occurs between the second and fourth days postpartum. It is minimized by proper positioning and good feeds. Check your positioning, and feed your baby often, paying close attention to proper position and latch. Ensure that she is finished feeding before she comes off the breast, by using breast compression (as described earlier on pp. 87-89) when necessary.

If your breasts are so full that the baby can't latch onto the breast, you may need to express a little milk to soften up the areola before you try to feed. You may want to do this in a warm bath or shower or after placing warm compresses on your breast. For relief of pain and pressure, you may want to do this between feeds as well.

Green cabbage leaves wrapped around your breasts for 15-20 minutes twice a day may help with the pain and pressure. Roll the leaves with a rolling pin if necessary, so the leaves can accommodate the shape of your breasts. You should stop when the symptoms resolve. You usually will need only 2-3 treatments.

If you cannot get your baby latched onto your breast despite the above interventions, pump your breasts and feed your baby the expressed milk until your baby is able to feed from your breast. If you don't have a high-quality pump, you can hand express the milk as described on p. 67. Pumping or expressing milk is important when the baby is not feeding at the breast so that your milk supply does not decrease.

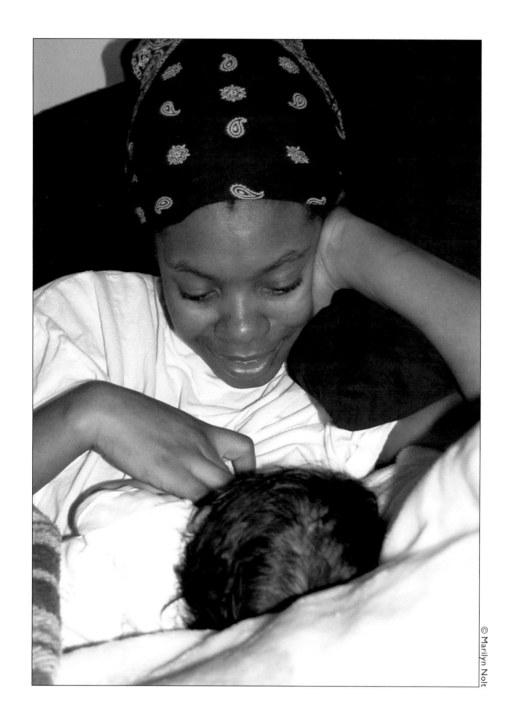

A Note about Colic and Frequent Feeding in the Coming Weeks —*CHECK POSITIONING:*

If your baby becomes uncomfortable with frequent crying spells associated with apparent gassiness or abdominal cramping in the following weeks or months, it may be a result of poor positioning at the breast. You may have never had ideal positioning and things were okay until now, or you may have slacked off on your positioning. Poor positioning causes the baby to feed less efficiently, and he is not able to extract the high-calorie hindmilk which comes during the latter part of the feed. The baby may gain well because the baby will get enough calories by getting a large enough volume of foremilk. The foremilk is higher in sugar and lower in fat than the hindmilk and can cause the baby to become gassy because of an overload of sugar. By not getting a high enough proportion of hindmilk, the baby needs to take in a larger volume to meet his calorie needs and feeds more frequently. The extra milk volume may lead to gastrointestinal discomfort. The frequent feeding may become overwhelming for you.

A correction in positioning allows for a proper latch and often brings about a happier baby and Mom. You may have the baby's head too far over to the breastfeeding side. Now that the baby is bigger, you may need to allow more room for his legs. An armed chair may push against his legs, incorrectly shifting his head position.

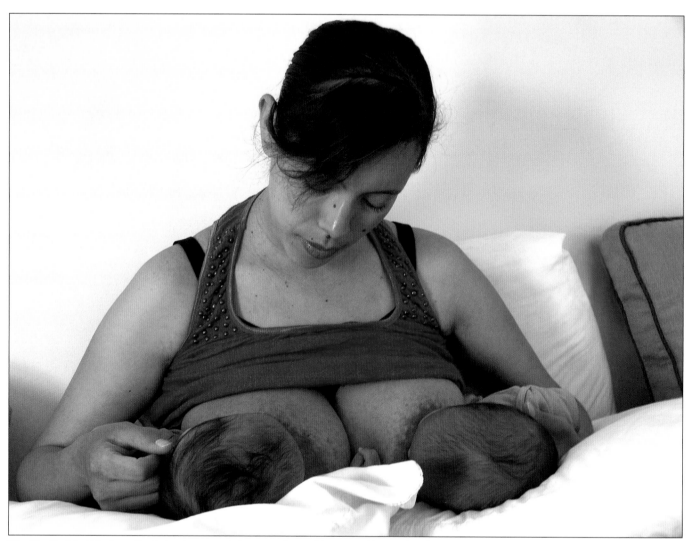

The "football hold" allows the twins to nurse at the same time without touching each other.

The Twin Experience

Breastfeeding twins can be very rewarding if the mom has the support she needs. Mom needs to be well nourished and cared for as she cares for her babies.

Positioning twins so that they can be nursed at the same time saves precious time. Notice the use of pillows in these photographs. Pillows support Mom's back and arms and allow the babies to be placed so that Mom does not have to fully support their weights.

Although it may be preferable to nurse two babies at the same time, it is uncommon to be able to feed twins at the same time from the start. If you find difficulty feeding your babies at the same time, feed each baby one at a time at first to learn the basics and each baby's unique feeding behavior.

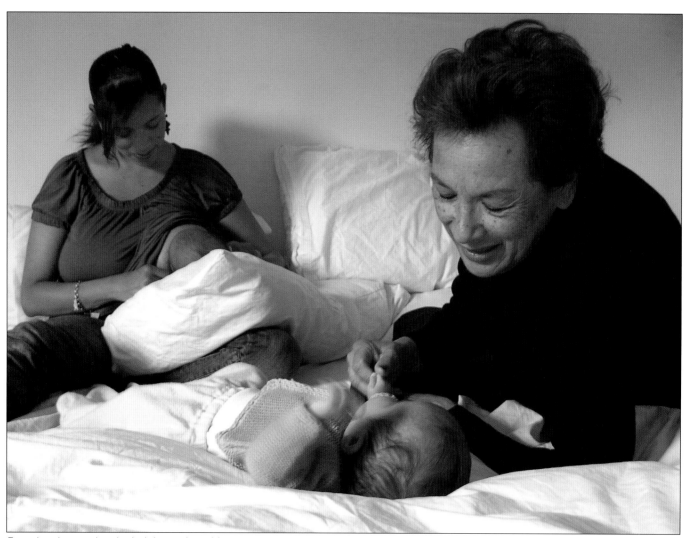

Extra hands ease the physical demands on Mom.

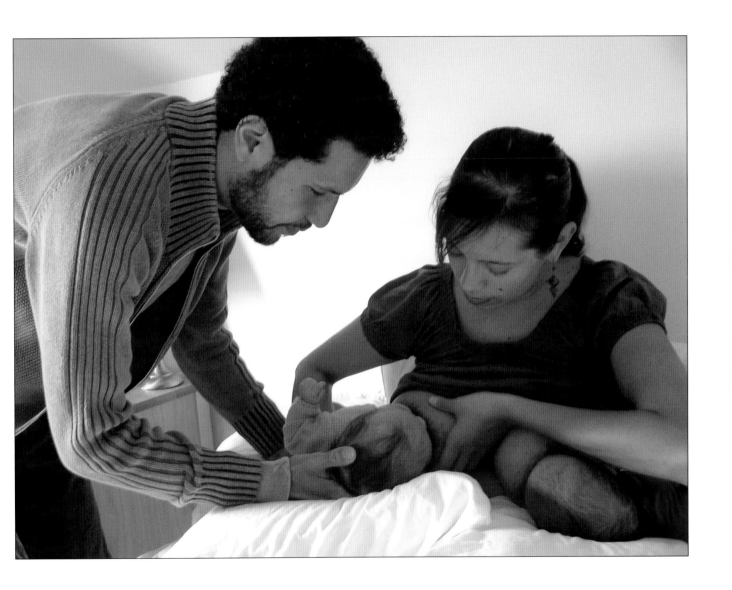

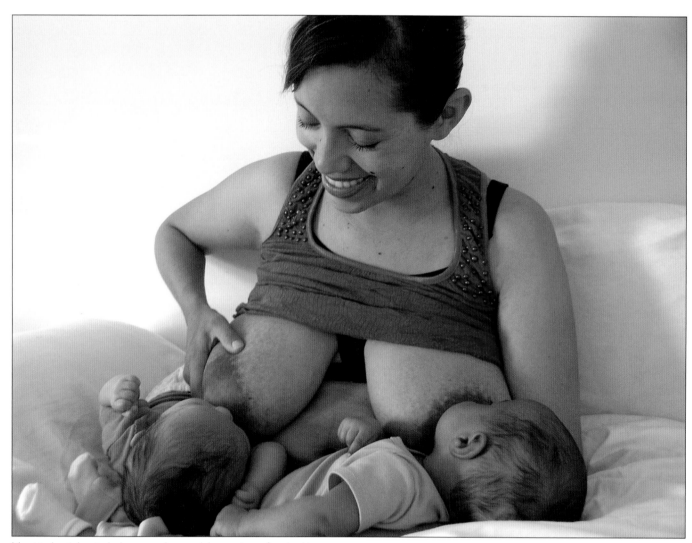

Most twins tolerate being very close or lying on top of each other.

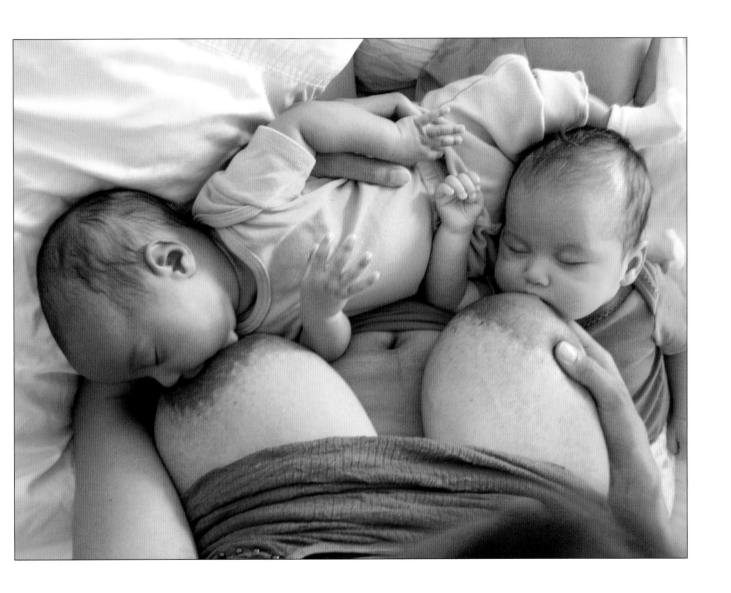

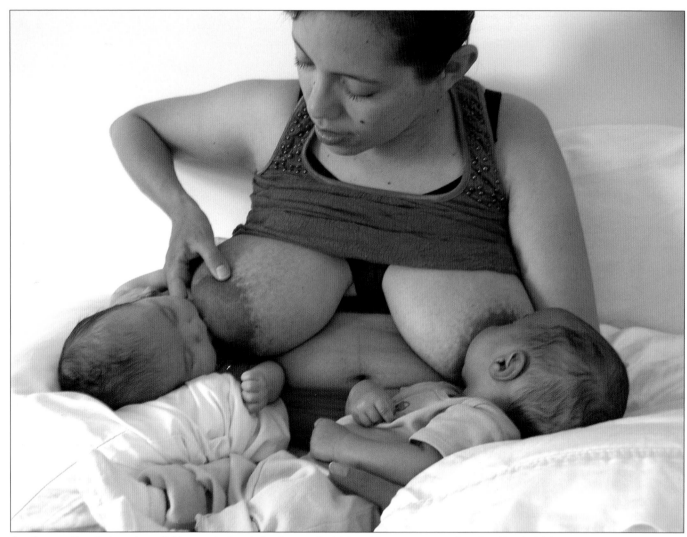

Another position that works well. Her son is already feeding comfortably as Mom encourages her daughter to latch.

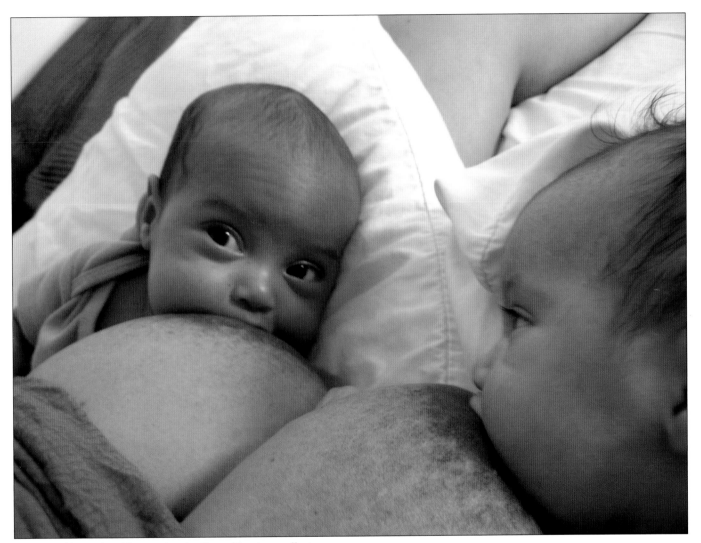

They are able to view Mom and each other without any effort.

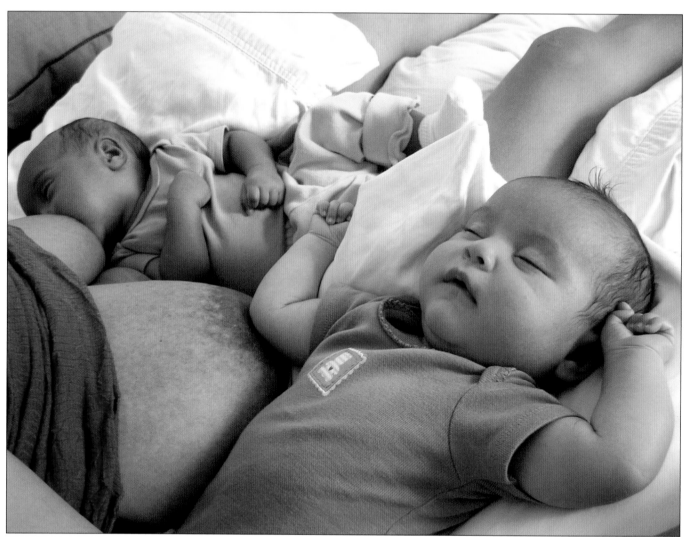

She is finished and satisfied while her brother leisurely finishes his feeding.

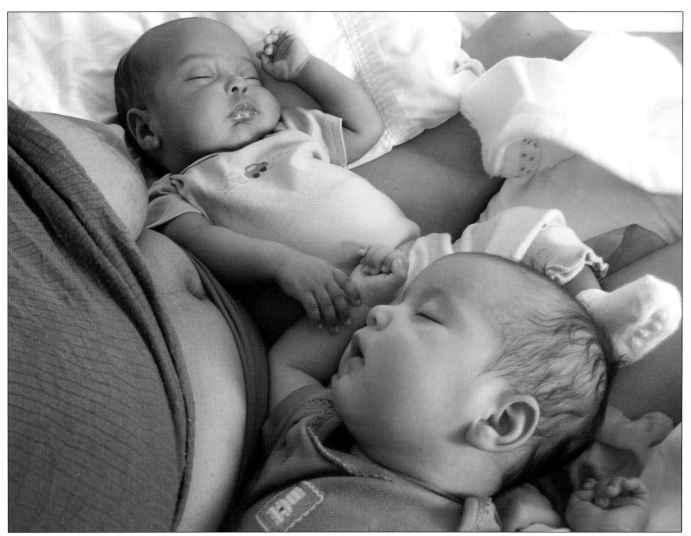

These nursing twins are content and satisfied after their feeds. They appear to be comforted by the closeness of their mom and each other.

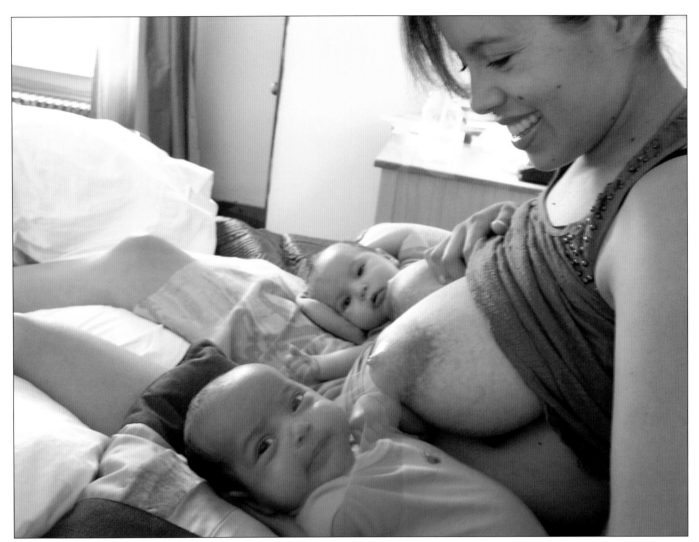

Happy babies at the breast are a source of pride and joy for Mom.

A Note about Breast Candida

Consider candida if you have breast or nipple pain after a period of pain-free nursing. Symptoms may include one or more of the following:

- Redness of your breast or nipple/areola. Redness is often not present so you should still consider candida even if there is no redness.
- Burning nipple or breast pain.
- Shooting pains through your breast during or between feeds.
- Blocked milk ducts that feel hard and painful to the touch.
- Achiness in your breasts.

You often may have only one of these symptoms early on in your candida infection. It is advisable to address the infection as early as possible.

Speak to your health care provider about your symptoms, and ask her to consider breast candida in her differential diagnosis if you feel it is a possibility. Because there is inconsistent knowledge about breast candida, it sometimes needs to be brought to your health care provider's attention.

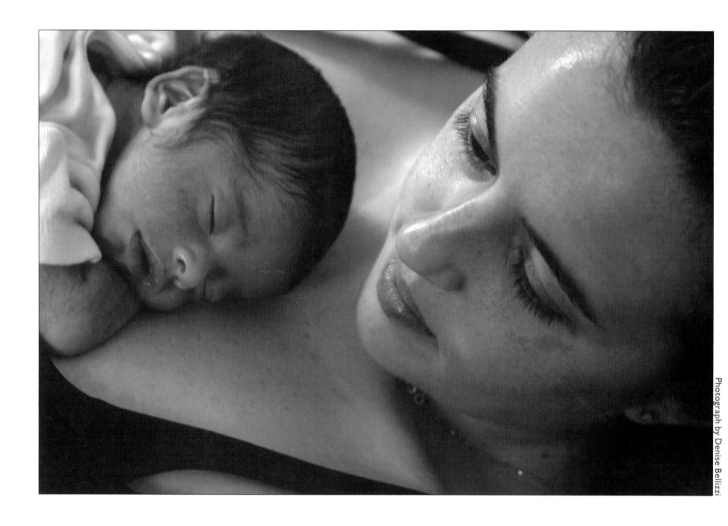

The Breastfeeding Relationship

The demands of breastfeeding ease greatly as the weeks go by, and it is best to take things one day at a time. Do not try to decide in the beginning how long you want to breastfeed. Often women become overwhelmed in the beginning and stop for fear of not being able "to keep this up." It is important to remember how much things change. The hard work you put in now will pay off in incredible ways that you can't possibly anticipate.

Describing what breastfeeding can do for you and your baby could fill the pages of this book (and is worth exploring). It is wonderful if breastfeeding comes easily; but if you are overwhelmed at first, understand that learning to breastfeed with comfort and joy is a process that often takes time— just as the benefits for you and your baby unfold over time.

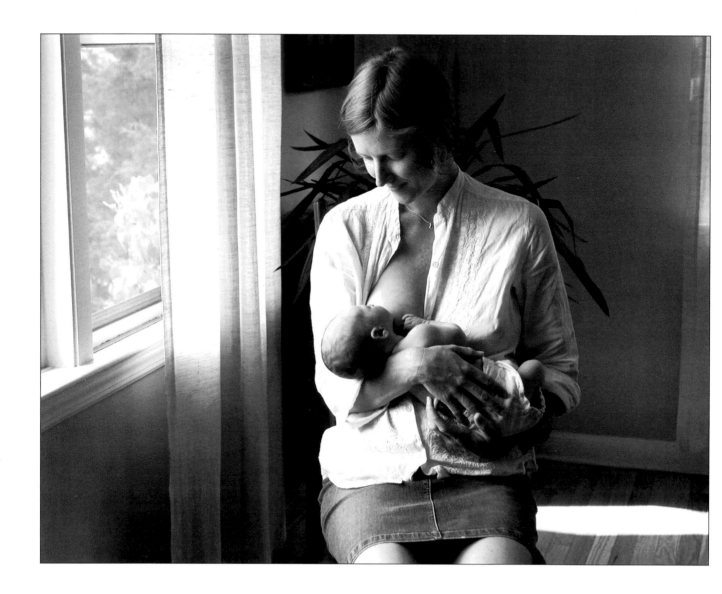

Breastfeeding Is Timeless

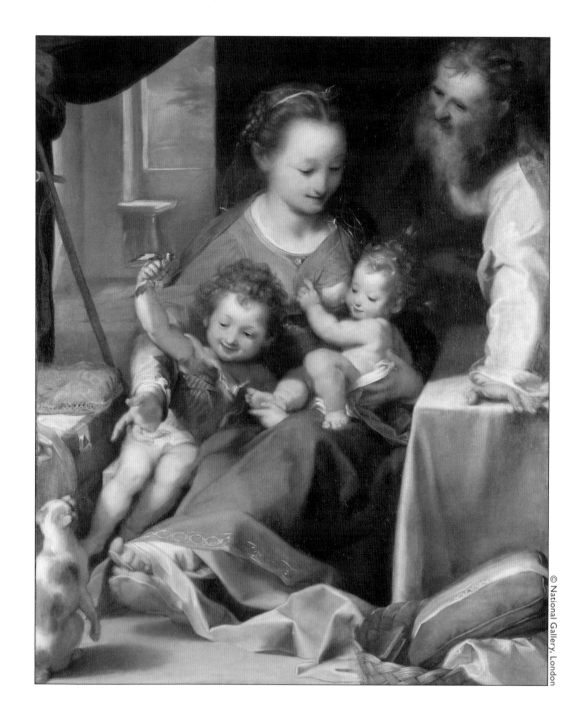

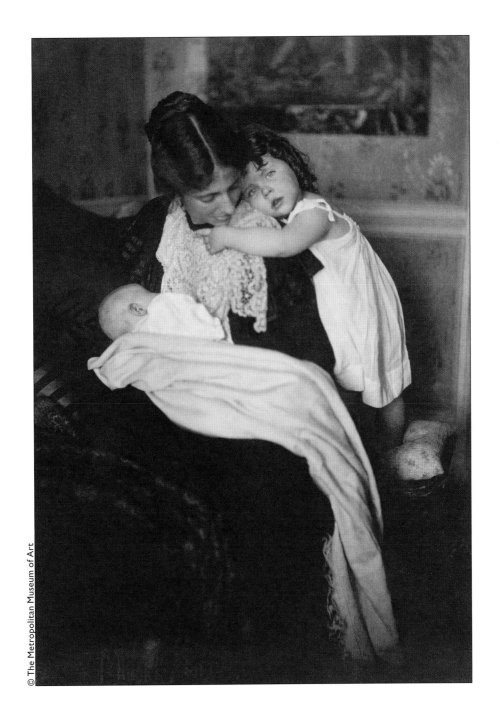

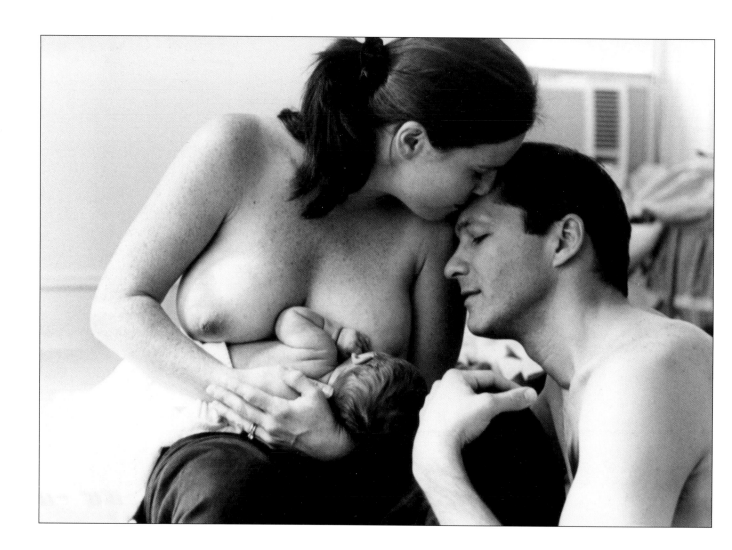

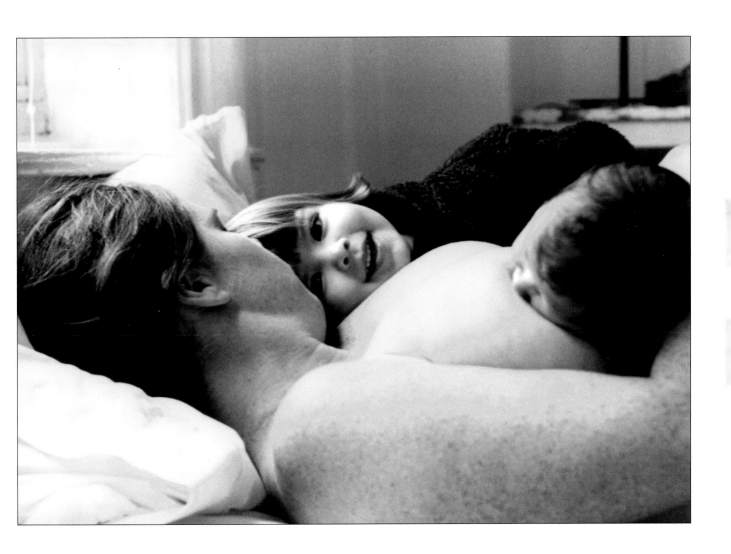

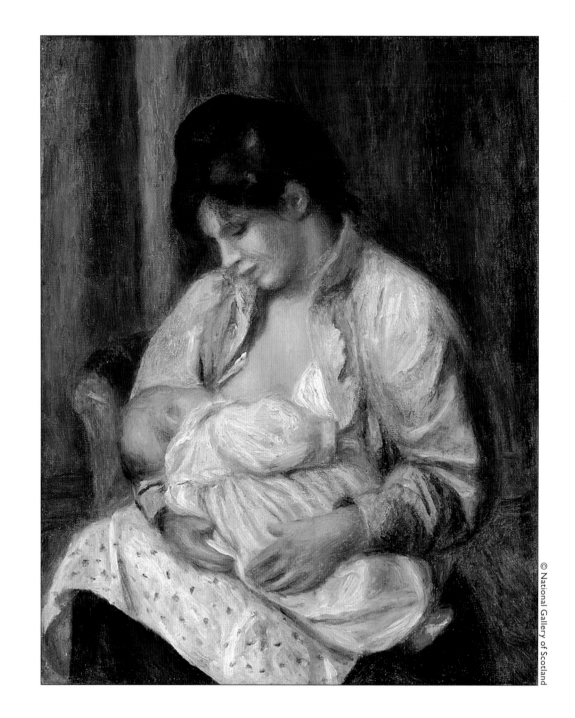

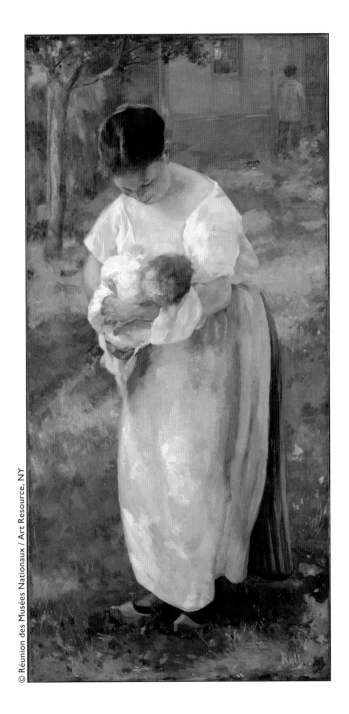

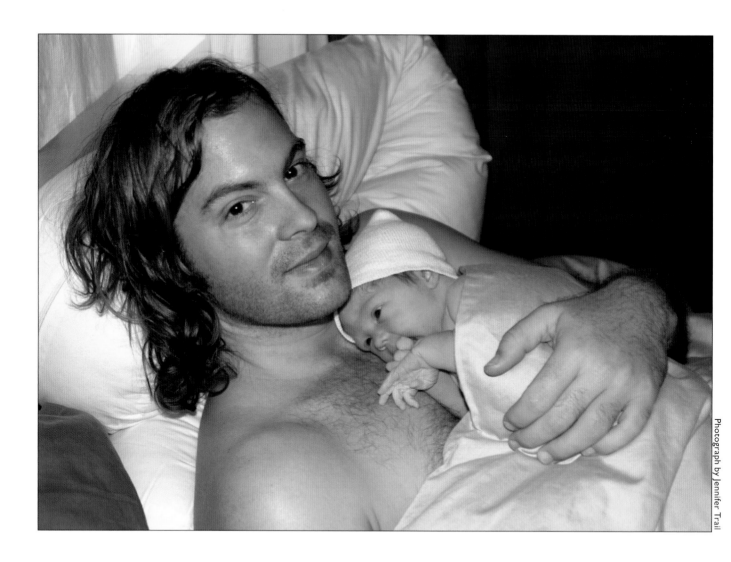

Photograph by Jennifer Trail

Appendix A

Moms Regulate Their Premature Babies' Skin Temperatures with Kangaroo Care

Continuous skin-to-skin contact between the premature baby and his mother is called Kangaroo Care. The premature baby is placed skin-to-skin with his mother and is covered with a diaper and blanket. What to do before, during and after Kangaroo Care is described in detail in *Kangaroo Care* (Ludington-Hoe 109-128).

The benefits of Kangaroo Care for the premature baby are well documented. It improves the premature baby's body temperature, heart rate, breathing patterns and oxygen saturation, weight and growth, sleep and alertness, emotional state, breastfeeding patterns, and bonding. Babies cry less and are discharged earlier from the hospital (Ludington-Hoe 67-84).

In her research, Dr. Ludington-Hoe specifically noted that mothers practicing Kangaroo Care unconsciously regulated their preemies' skin temperatures to be in the correct range by adjusting their own skin temperatures. In addition, when a mother was told that her baby was getting cold, her breast temperature rose in response, increasing her baby's skin temperature (Ludington-Hoe 29-30).

She writes the following account of her observations in her book *Kangaroo Care* (Ludington-Hoe 29-30).

> One of my first and perhaps most fascinating findings was that mothers unconsciously regulate their premies' skin temperatures by changing their own temperature in response. When we monitored the skin temperature of mothers' breasts, we found that it increased when their premies began to cool, and dropped when their babies warmed up.
>
> After observing this phenomenon with twelve mother-infant pairs, my research associates Carol Thompson, Joan Swinth, and I wondered if telling a woman that her infant was becoming cold would hasten her regulating her own temperature. We decided to give it a try. Standing behind a mother, Carol told her, "Looks like your baby is becoming a little cold." Within two minutes, her breast temperature shot up two full degrees centigrade (about 3.6 degrees Fahrenheit). That brought the premie's skin temperature up.
>
> Once the baby's skin temperature approached the upper limit, I told this mother, "He's warm enough now." And sure enough, over the next two minutes, her breast temperature fluctuated one to two degrees centigrade to keep the baby at a steady, normal temperature. We call this unconscious regulation "maternal-neonatal thermal synchrony."

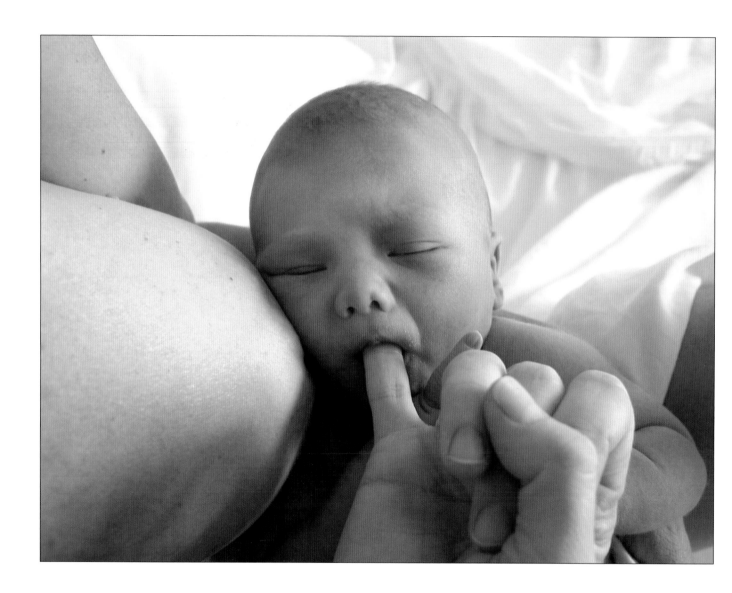

Appendix B

Things to Consider If You Are Reading This Before Having Your Baby

A note about medication during labor and delivery

Maternal drugs during labor and delivery can affect your baby's alertness. A medicated newborn is usually less alert than an unmedicated newborn. A less alert baby likely will be less active at the breast. The medications also can directly affect the baby's ability to coordinate suckling at the breast.

The effect of medication on a newborn baby is clearly seen in Dr. Righard's video, entitled *Delivery Self Attachment*. This video is based on Dr. Righard's study published in *The Lancet*. In his study, most newborns from a medicated birth were too drowsy to be able to suckle. In contrast, the unmedicated babies were able to self-attach. The most consistently correct suckling and self-attachment patterns were seen in the unmedicated babies where there was no interference with the babies and moms at birth. The babies were immediately placed on the mothers' abdomens and not temporarily taken away for hospital routines such as bathing and measuring.

The difficulties sometimes caused by medication can certainly be overcome. However, avoidance of medication, if possible, can make breastfeeding easier and allows for the gift of a more alert newborn.

If you want to avoid medication during labor, you should communicate your wishes to your obstetrician or midwife. You may also want to consider having a doula, a woman trained to provide you with the emotional and physical support that can ease the pain of labor and thus minimize the need for medication.

You can also speak to your obstetrician or midwife about delaying the hospital routines at birth so that the first hour or so can be devoted to uninterrupted contact between you and your baby. This optimizes the environment for your baby to begin breastfeeding well from birth. A good first feed can establish a good foundation for breastfeeding.

A note about circumcision

Circumcision is an elective procedure and can temporarily affect your baby boy's activity. If you are struggling with breastfeeding, circumcision can be the last straw and have a negative impact. If you have made the decision to circumcise your baby, the procedure can be delayed. It does not have to take place in the hospital, allowing you and your baby time to settle in together in the days following the birth. You can research mohels in your area who do both religious and nonreligious circumcisions.

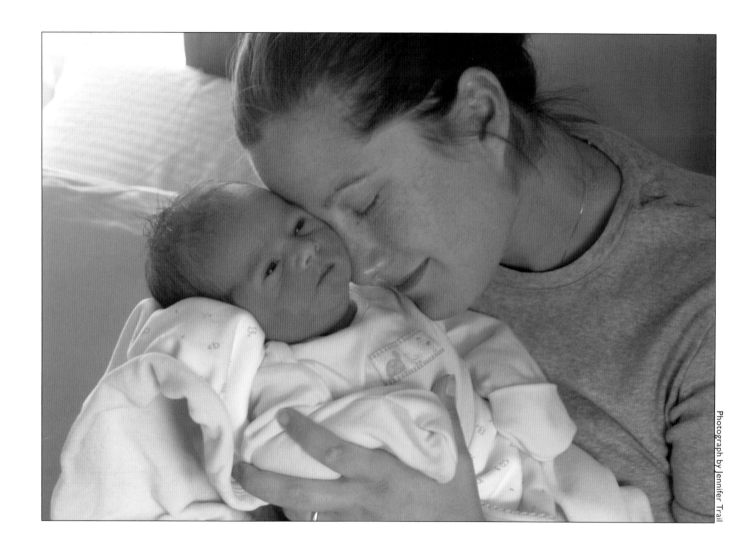

Photograph by Jennifer Trail

Appendix C
Special Situations and Conditions that May Challenge You

Women are often told there is something wrong with the anatomy of their breasts or their babies' mouths or suckling patterns. They are told their breasts are too big or their nipples are too large or inverted. They are also told their babies' mouths are too small or they don't open wide enough or their lips aren't flanged out enough at the breast, or they are tongue-tied. They are also told that their babies are making the wrong sounds when they are breastfeeding. You should not assume these statements are indicative of an impending problem. Most babies, despite these conditions, can breastfeed without difficulty. Paying close attention to the position and latch is more important in these situations because it can affect the challenges each of these situations may impose. Most of the challenges, if present, resolve themselves a few days after the birth if you pay close attention to the baby's latch. In the case of tongue-tie, most babies do not have problems with breastfeeding. For those who do, your doctor or ENT specialist can snip the frenulum. It is important to remember, babies and their mothers are always unique pairs, and nature intended for breastfeeding to work well without an anatomy prescription.

Women are often given incorrect information about **breast surgery's** impact on breastfeeding. It is most important not to make the assumption that you will not be able to breastfeed. Pay close attention to your position and latch to help the baby get the milk you do have.

Polycystic ovary syndrome (PCOS) is another condition about which women are often given incorrect information. Sometimes women are told they have PCOS without a definitive diagnosis. The breastfeeding experience in a woman with PCOS is unpredictable. Women's milk supplies vary greatly. It is important not to eliminate the hope of breast-feeding. Again, pay close attention to your position and latch to maximize your baby's intake of breastmilk.

The recommendations for **increasing your milk supply** are many and varied and beyond the scope of this book. The simplest area that can be addressed is your diet. You should pay close attention to maintaining adequate fluid, calories, protein, and healthy fat intake. A lactation aid is a very useful tool for increasing your milk supply (Appendix E).

Women are often challenged physically and emotionally when they go **back to work**. The increased demands of their jobs and the separation from their babies can impact their milk supplies. One often-overlooked intervention is to allow more physical contact with your baby when you are not at work. You can provide skin-to-skin contact as described in this book; and you can wear your baby, bathe with your baby, and sleep near your baby if you wish. It is interesting to note that the energy field of your heart has been measured and found to radiate at least 3 feet around you. Thus, it can be experienced by your baby sleeping near you just as your baby experienced it during your pregnancy.

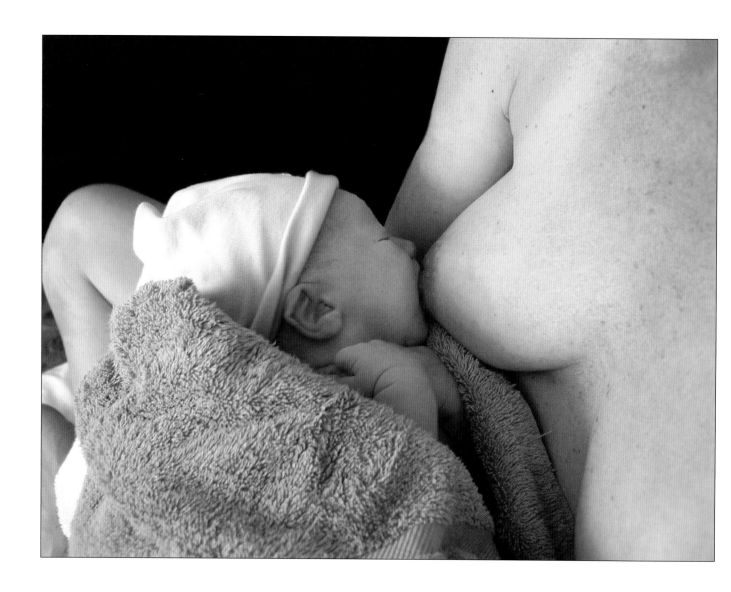

Appendix D
Babies with Special Needs and Premature Babies and Jaundice

The specific care of premature babies, babies with special needs, and babies with jaundice is beyond the scope of this book. Please refer to *Bestfeeding: How to Breastfeed Your Baby* and *The Ultimate Breastfeeding Book of Answers* for more detailed discussions. Remember the importance of skin-to-skin contact in every situation. If you have to be separated from your baby for medical reasons, understand the challenges presented and try to minimize the time apart, if possible.

When you are allowed time together, try to have skin-to-skin contact. Pump your breasts to maintain your milk supply and provide nourishment for your baby.

In cases where there is a concern regarding jaundice, it is important to understand the benefits of good feeds facilitated by the correct latch. The increased breastmilk helps the baby to eliminate the bilirubin, present in jaundice, more efficiently. Jaundice can also be a normal finding in a healthy baby and, in this case, is termed physiological jaundice.

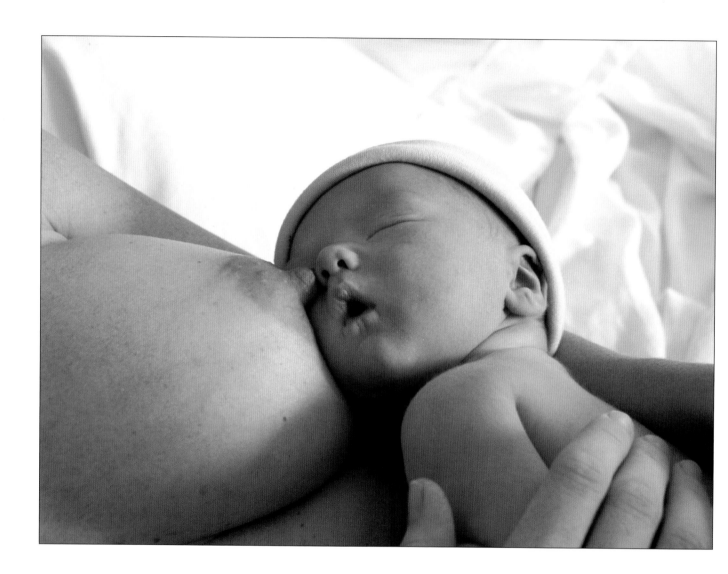

Appendix E
Different Modalities for Feeding Expressed Breastmilk

Breastfeeding is not more difficult than bottle-feeding. In fact, a baby's vital signs reveal that it takes less energy to breastfeed as is revealed by a lower heart rate and respiratory rate. Thus, we do not need to give a baby special bottles to slow the flow and make the baby "work harder" to be more like breastfeeding as women are often told. A mother usually can assess what bottle or nipple her baby should use based on her own good sense about the baby's comfort level.

In my practice, I do not generally advocate cup feeding or syringe feeding unless there is a medical indication because it forces the baby to drink, utilizing a feeding mechanism that is quite unnatural and unlike babies' natural pleasurable suckling instincts. I also do not usually recommend syringe feeding with the finger, or finger feeding with a feeding tube attached to the finger and connected to a milk reservoir. Finger feeding allows for suckling, unlike the cup, but it is at great energy expenditure for the parents if it goes on more than a day or two. If the breastfeeding problem has not been solved or addressed, the fatigue and frustration only increase with time. A bottle is easier and in this case, easier is better because the baby will return to the breast. We don't want women giving up breastfeeding because it is too hard to finger feed or cup feed. However, finger feeding can be used to prepare the baby to take the breast; it should not be used as a substitute for the bottle. If the baby is 'refusing' the breast, the mother finger feeds for 30-60 seconds and then tries the baby on the breast.

Some babies need to be fed with feeding tubes or special bottles for medical reasons that make it impossible for them to suckle. **Lactation aids** are used when the baby has the ability to suckle but there is a milk supply issue. The feeding tube of a lactation aid can be inserted into a milk reservoir and attached to the mother's nipple/areola when a mother is trying to initiate (i.e., adoption) or augment a truly insufficient milk supply. The suckling action of the baby increases the mother's production of hormones responsible for milk synthesis and production. The baby simultaneously gets milk from the breast and from the milk reservoir.

The Haberman bottle is a unique bottle. It was designed to be used for babies with cleft palate. The mechanics of feeding from the Haberman bottle involve pumping without suckling and do not allow the baby to create a vacuum. Making it impossible to create a vacuum is appropriate and necessary for a baby with cleft palate and was a breakthrough in the care of these babies. However, it is not appropriate for a term baby without any medical problems. Promotion of this bottle includes the statement that breastfeeding is primarily pumping, and bottle-feeding is primarily suckling. The incorrect conclusion is drawn that because the Haberman only involves pumping, it is more like breastfeeding than a regular bottle. In fact, the baby is not able to create a vacuum and suckle at all with the Haberman, and thus it is less like breastfeeding than a regular bottle.

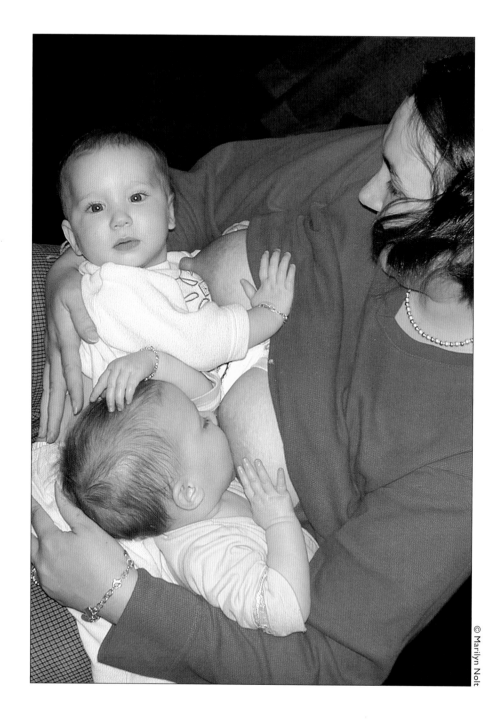

Appendix E (cont.)

The Haberman bottle is currently used for a variety of other reasons such as slowing the milk flow with a dial so the baby has to "work harder to strengthen his suck." Sucking is a reflex, and the baby should not need to be forced to work harder in order to strengthen his suck and get food. However, slowing the milk flow may be necessary for medical or other reasons.

A truly weak suck is rare and is observed whether the baby is feeding from the breast or bottle or sucking on an adult's finger. It is usually temporary and will become stronger with time without outside intervention or special bottles or nipples. If there is a neurological issue, a baby's suck may be weakened. Often these issues resolve with time, but working with a cranial sacral therapist experienced with newborns can facilitate the development of the baby's ability to suck efficiently. A neurological problem is not resolved with special bottles or nipples.

Implementation of the UNICEF/WHO Baby Friendly Hospital Initiative involves 10 steps that promote and support breastfeeding. Step 9 states, "Give no pacifiers or artificial nipples to breastfeeding infants." I do not believe providing a baby with expressed breastmilk from a bottle violates the intention of this code. This step is addressing the routine use of offering pacifiers and bottles to breastfed babies. Routine use is not supportive of breastfeeding. However, when a baby is not able to feed at the breast for days or weeks for whatever reason, bottles of expressed breastmilk do not impair a baby's ability to later breastfeed.

Bibliography

Arms, Suzanne. *Immaculate Deception II Myth, Magic and Birth*. Berkeley, California: Celestial Arts, 1996.

Delivery Self Attachment. Righard, Lennart and Kittie Frantz. Videocassette. Sunland, CA: Geddes Productions, 1992.

Fisher, Chloe and Sally Inch. "Nipple confusion— who is confused?" *The Journal of Pediatrics*. 1996; 129(1): 174.

Ludington-Hoe, Susan M., and Susan K. Golant. *Kangaroo Care*. New York: Bantam Books, 1993.

Newman, Jack. *Is My Baby Getting Enough?* Printed and written by Jack Newman, revised January 2005.

Newman, Jack and Teresa Pitman. *The Ultimate Breastfeeding Book of Answers Revised and Updated*. New York: Three Rivers Press, 2006.

Odent, Michel. *Birth Reborn*. Illinois: Livingstone, 1994.

Renfrew, Mary, Chloe Fisher and Suzanne Arms. *Bestfeeding: How to Breastfeed Your Baby*. Berkeley, California: Ten Speed Press, 2004.

Righard, Lennart, and Margaret O. Alade. "Effect of Delivery Room Routines on Success of First Breast-feed." *The Lancet*. 1990; 336: 1105-1107.

Credits

All photographs by Laura Keegan unless otherwise credited.

P. 120   Fedrico Barocci
The Madonna and Child with Saint Joseph and the Infant Baptist ('La Madonna del Gatto'), about 1575
Oil on canvas, 112.7 x 92.7 cm
Bequeathed by Revd Holwell Carr, 1831
(NG 29)
© National Gallery, London

P. 121   Gertrude Käsebier (1852-1934)
Family Group, 1902
Platinum print, 19.6 x 13.7 cm
The Metropolitan Museum of Art, Alfred Stieglitz Collection, 1933
(33.43.370)
© The Metropolitan Museum of Art

P. 124   Pierre-Auguste Renoir
A Woman Nursing a Child, about 1894
Oil on canvas, 41.2 x 32.5 cm
(NG 2230)
© National Gallery of Scotland

P. 125   Alfred Roll (1846-1919)
The Wetnurse Louise Cattel
Oil on canvas, 157 x 74 cm
Musee des Beaux-Arts, Lille, France
(ART173020)
© Réunion des Musées Nationaux / Art Resource, NY

Design and layout by Jennifer Trail (www.intrinsicaudiovisual.com).

About the Author

Laura Keegan is a Family Nurse Practitioner (FNP) in clinical practice since 1988. Her formal education includes a Bachelor of Science With Highest Honors majoring in Physiology from the University of California at Davis. Her nursing education includes two Master of Science degrees from Pace University.

Laura's clinical practice in New York State began in 1986 as an RN at Montefiore Medical Center in the Bronx. She began her work as an FNP at the Institute for Urban Family Health in Manhattan in 1988, and later with the Peekskill Area Health Center and Riverside Pediatrics in Croton-on-Hudson, New York. She maintains a holistic solo private family practice in Dutchess County, New York.

In her career, Laura has helped hundreds of breastfeeding women who came to her with significant problems and hundreds of others who she helped to get started in establishing a comfortable breastfeeding relationship. She has attended many conferences on breastfeeding and lactation and reviewed dozens of breastfeeding videos and books in order to learn as much as she could about breastfeeding. However, her best teachers have been moms and babies, and this book is drawn from her years of work with breastfeeding women. Laura views every mom and baby as a unique pair of individuals that she is honored to care for during this sacred time.

More information about Laura and her practice can be found on the web at www.lifeforcefamilyhealth.com or www.laurakeegan.com.

Laura is the mother of four children, all breastfed.